Glaucoma
How To Save Your Sight

ACKNOWLEDGEMENTS

Gratefully we acknowledge assistance for Portuguese-English translation by Dr Gustavo Muradas-Reiss and for development of the manuscript for publication as a book by Simon Bakker, Kugler Publications.

Glaucoma
How To Save Your Sight

Written by

**Ivan Goldberg
Remo Susanna Jr.**

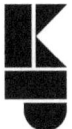

Kugler Publications/Amsterdam/The Netherlands

ISBN 978-90-6299-242-3

Kugler Publications
P.O. Box 20538
1001 NM Amsterdam, The Netherlands
www.kuglerpublications.com

© 2015 Kugler Publications, Amsterdam, The Netherlands
All rights reserved. No part of this book may be translated or reproduced in any form by print, photoprint, microfilm, or any other means without prior written permission of the publisher.

Kugler Publications is an imprint of SPB Academic Publishing bv, P.O. Box 20538, 1001 NM Amsterdam, The Netherlands

Cover design: Willem Driebergen, Rijnsburg, The Netherlands

Table of Content

Preface 7

1. Introduction 9

2. Improved care 11

3. The seven 'sins' in glaucoma 13

4. Glaucoma treatment 61

5. Most common myths in glaucoma 89

6. Other forms of glaucoma worth knowing about . . 102

7. Glaucoma and cataract together 121

Appendix 1: How to instil eye drops 125

Appendix 2: How to do the best-possible
visual field test 127

Further reading 131

About the authors 133

Frequently asked questions 137

Index key words 141

Preface

Glaucoma is infamous as 'the sneak thief of sight': the most common types give no warning they are slowly, progressively destroying a person's vision. Because usually the vision at first is affected to the side, patients notice little, if anything. By the time an individual realizes something is wrong, there may have been considerable damage.

Why write a book about it? And why dedicate it to all patients with glaucoma, to their relatives and friends, to the general community as well as to ophthalmologists, other doctors and eye health care practitioners who wish to be familiar with management of this group of diseases?

Undisturbed, glaucoma blinds people. It respects neither gender nor education; it ignores wealth and privilege. We have no cure for it and we cannot reverse the damage that it has caused. Glaucoma affects about 2% of people over 40 years of age. It is not rare. It is the commonest cause of irreversible and preventable visual disability everywhere.

But most of the time we can control it. Successful protection of vision depends in part on how much damage has been done when first detected and how aggressive the disease is for an individual patient. So the earlier glaucoma is diagnosed, the less damage that has been caused, the better the long-term outlook.

Early detection requires informed communities whose members seek eye examinations as well as knowledgeable and appropriately equipped eye health care professionals who recognize subtle warning signs and arrange timely ophthalmological confirmation and initiation of effective treatment. This requires access to a worthwhile health system.

Even in developed societies, about 50% of patients with glaucoma have not been diagnosed and are not on treatment. Half of these undiagnosed people have been seen by an eye health care practitioner in the last two years.

We wish to enlighten our readers with quality information to minimize visual disability from glaucoma.

Ivan Goldberg
Remo Susanna Jr.

1. Introduction

How miraculous is the ability to see? As the organ of sight, the eye captures light, focuses it and begins its transformation into nerve impulses along the visual pathways enabling visual perception by the brain. The eye focuses far and near and in between objects too; it notes movement, direction, brightness, colour, distance, contrast and the brain compensates for head and body movements so we know where we are in relation to what we are viewing. Simultaneously we attach relative importance and relevance to what is around us, so perception and interpretation proceed alongside one another (Fig. 1).

On a safari in Africa, guides display an uncanny ability to locate camouflaged animals through training and concentration. The visual system is capable of training, of responding to needs, to optimize specific functions. Indeed the eye is an integral part of the brain itself. That is why, with current technologies, any damage in the optic nerve is irreversible. Perhaps one day stem cells will enable regeneration.

Directly and indirectly our sight influences all aspects of our lives. That is why we fear blindness almost as much as we fear death and why we invest so much emotion into our eyes.

In this book we wish to guide the reader, whether patient or eye care health worker, on how to minimize visual disability from the glaucomas.

Glaucoma: How to Save Your Sight!

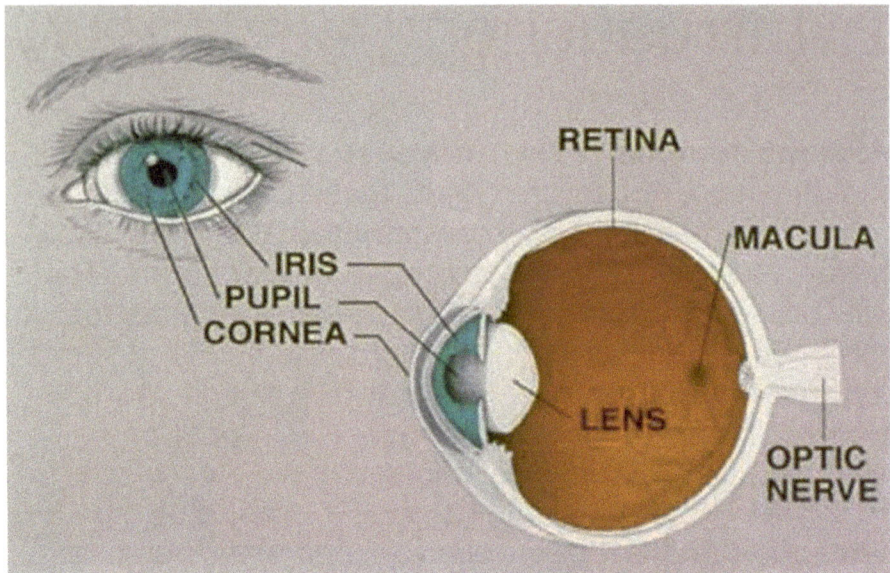

Fig. 1. Light passes through the cornea (the front window of the eye) and enters through the pupil (the aperture formed by the coloured part of the eye, the iris). It is focused by the lens onto the retina. Central vision (reading, writing, recognising faces) is created at the macula. Carrying the messages of sight, nerve fibres from the retina meet at the back of the eye where they turn through 90 degrees to exit, forming the head of the optic nerve through which they pass back to the seeing part of the brain. It is where they turn and exit that glaucoma kills these nerves, thereby breaking the essential link between eye and brain. That is how it damages sight.

2. Improved care

How can we explain the 2013 report from Sweden that in a city where renowned eye doctors in a famous university cared for glaucoma patients, 16.4% became blind in both eyes and 42.2% blind in one eye, of whom 20% also had severe visual damage in their fellow (better) eye?

This is remarkably similar to information reported in 1965 from Olmstead County in the United States where over many years, 14% of glaucoma patients became blind in both eyes and a further 27% became blind in one eye.

After 42 years of progress in disease diagnosis, in assessment of risk factors, in advances in eye drop medications, laser techniques and surgical approaches, these reported blindness rates are almost unchanged. Why?

How might we improve this situation? Ongoing scientific advances and improved information resources will help. So will improved communication between ophthalmologists and between all eye care workers with one another and with the community. If patients were to be more knowledgeable and increasingly involved in their care, we believe it would make a real difference for the better. We hope this book will enhance understanding and promote efficient interaction between patients and their doctors, to assist vision protection with improved monitoring of the disease and more effective treatment.

Focal Points

- Glaucoma is increasingly common with increasing age and varies between different ethnic groups. It is ten times more likely if there is a family history.

- With adequate care, for most people, glaucoma should be able to be controlled.

- There are "seven deadly sins", which can contribute to visual disability from glaucoma:
    1. Non-diagnosis: failure to have regular eye checks, especially with a family history; failure to check the health of the optic nerve and to rely excessively on eye pressure measurements.
    2. Failure to recognize progressive damage: this needs regular review with adequate use of visual fields and optic disc assessment technologies.
    3. Failure to diagnose accurately the type of glaucoma to guide accurate management.
    4. Failure to stage disease severity accurately: the more severe the damage, the more aggressive the treatment needs to be.
    5. Insufficient reduction in the eye pressure: the more severe the damage, the greater the eye pressure reduction needs to be.
    6. Delay in onset of treatment: if there is damage, it must be recognized and treatment started to provide protection.
    7. Patient non-adherence or non-perseverance with treatment.

3. The seven 'sins' in glaucoma

Glaucomas are more common than we think. While one in 200 people has glaucoma at the age of 40 years, by 80, it is one in ten. While glaucomas have no gender bias overall, **affecting men and women equally**, the angle closure varieties do like the ladies a bit more.

Variations between different groups of people are fascinating and point to a strong genetic influence: the open-angle glaucomas are more common in African-derived peoples, the angle closures being more common in Chinese, other Asian and Inuit populations. Glaucomas associated with pseudoexfoliation are more common in Nordic groups and Russian Jews. More than people elsewhere, the Japanese and Koreans suffer from glaucoma damage with eye pressures that often lie within the usual range found in the community. What is important is that all groups of humans suffer from the full range of glaucomas.

Besides age and ethnicity, family history is very important. If a person has a first-degree relative with glaucoma (mother, father, brother or sister), their own risk increases ten-fold. Glaucomas are also more common in individuals who suffer from migraine, cold hands and feet in winter, diabetes, short-sightedness, high blood pressure, those who smoke and those who have had to use steroid-type medications for long periods.

As far as we know, Hippocrates (460-377 BC), one of the fathers of modern Western medicine, was the first to describe glaucoma. He featured a disease glazing the pupil in a blue-green hue, leading to blindness. 'Glaucoma' derives from the ancient Greek word Γλαὐκος, which means 'blue-green' colour.

Four centuries later, Celsius believed glaucoma affected the crystalline (focusing) lens of the eye. It took almost two millennia for cataract ('cloudy lens') to be separated from glaucoma.

In 1835, Mackenzie linked glaucoma with intra-ocular pressure (IOP). For many people, glaucoma remains synonymous with a raised IOP, even though we know eye pressure does NOT characterize the condition. People suffer glaucoma damage to their optic nerves (the essential link between the eye and the brain); reducing IOP has a high chance of slowing or halting the disease, but 30% of Caucasians, 80% of Koreans and 90% of Japanese with glaucoma have never had elevated IOP measured. This makes diagnosis more challenging and may lead to glaucoma being missed, with possibly nasty results.

Losing vision from glaucoma is tragic. It should be avoidable for most, but unfortunately not all patients. When it occurs, as in most air crashes this disaster may follow a combination of misperceptions and oversights, each contributing differently to the final result. Sometimes the disease is relentless no matter what is done; sometimes it deceives the clinician as much as the patient. What are the most common misperceptions

3. Setting the scene for the seven 'sins'

and oversights? In other words, what are the most common 'sins' in glaucoma management?

3.1 Sin one: Non-diagnosis in glaucoma

Members of the community contribute to this sin by complacency, taking their good eye sight for granted and not arranging to have routine eye assessments. Even more so, people with a family history of glaucoma need to be seen themselves every couple of years after the age of 35 years.

Added to this is the persisting myth that anyone with an eye pressure less than 21 millimetres of mercury (mmHg) does not have glaucoma and need not be concerned. We know one-third of Caucasians with glaucoma never have IOP over 21 mmHg. **Measuring eye pressure alone is a terrible way to diagnose glaucoma. An eye check MUST include a careful assessment of the optic nerve at the back of the eye** and then if necessary, include a visual field test.

Eye pressure is a major risk factor for glaucoma: the higher it is, the greater the risk. But eye pressure levels are NOT synonymous with a glaucoma diagnosis. Not for many years has 'increased' IOP been part of the definition of glaucoma.

Raised eye pressures (above 'usual' levels) can be found without glaucoma damage - although high pressure increases risk as mentioned. People with higher than usual pressures but without other signs of glaucoma damage are called 'ocular hypertensives'. They are at increased risk of developing glaucoma. In turn, glaucoma damage can be found with 'usual' eye pressures. Sometimes people in this situation

3. Setting the scene for the seven 'sins'

are diagnosed as having 'low-tension' or 'normal-pressure' glaucoma. This may be misleading, as there is no evidence that patients in this situation have a different disease or need different treatment from other glaucoma sufferers.

Rather glaucoma is defined as a progressive optic neuropathy (disease process of the optic nerve) characterized by death of the nerve fibres carrying the essential messages of sight from the eye to the brain. When damaged by glaucoma, this connection is increasingly affected. Nerve fibre death is seen as paleness and erosion of the optic nerve structures and the nerve fibre layer of the retina.

At birth, each eye has about 1,200,000 nerve fibres linking it to the brain. It is very much akin to an old fashioned electric wire cable. As individual nerves are killed, like wires being cut, less information can be transmitted: a partly cut cable cannot carry instructions reliably from a wall light switch to the ceiling light.

Whereas in developed countries about 50% of glaucoma patients are undiagnosed, in developing nations that figure may be well over 90%. When many of these undiagnosed patients are finally discovered, tragically, the glaucoma is often advanced.

So how is eye pressure measured? Most commonly used is the current 'gold standard', applanation tonometry, usually using the device developed in the 1950s by a Swiss glaucoma specialist, Hans Goldmann. It is fitted to a slit lamp (bio-microscope) and determines IOP by measuring the force needed to flatten ('applanate') a very precise small area of the cornea (window of the eye). This force allows the internal eye pressure to be calculated (Figs. 2 and 3).

Another important measure that needs to be done at least once is the thickness of the central cornea, measured by ultrasound and known as pachymetry. For applanation to be accurate, central corneal thickness needs to be within a normal range (520-540 microns). If a person has inherited a thicker than usual cornea,

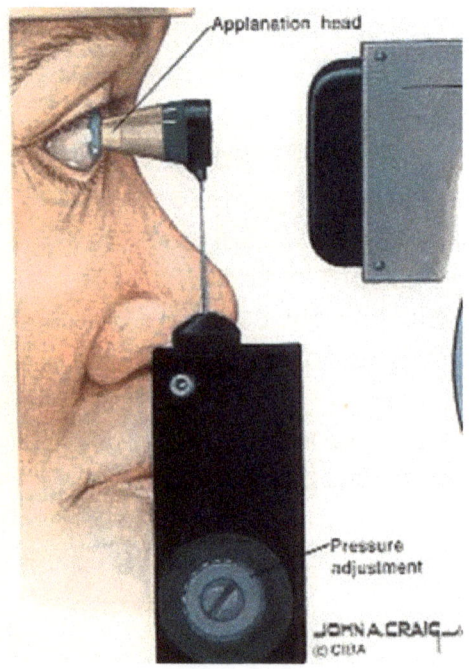

Fig. 2. Goldmann tonometer head applied gently to the front surface of the cornea and viewed through the slit-lamp biomicroscope. The eye health worker instils anaesthetic drops for comfort and fluorescein, which when illuminated with a cobalt-crystal blue light, highlights the circle of contact. Within the tonometer head is a bi-prism that splits this circular image into two semi-circles. Adjusting the dial varies the tension applied to the cornea, causing more or less flattening ('applanation') of the corneal surface. When the two semi-circles just overlap, the eye pressure is able to be read off the tonometer dial.

3. Setting the scene for the seven 'sins'

the applanation tonometer over-reads: the measured eye pressure is higher than the real level. This may be reassuring. Conversely, if the cornea is significantly thinner than usual, the tonometer will under-read: the measured eye pressure is lower than the real level. This may be falsely reassuring.

Laser surgery to the cornea at any time in one's life may thin the cornea and lead the tonometer significantly and forever to underestimate eye pressure. If you have ever had laser to your eyes, you must remember to inform your ophthalmologist.

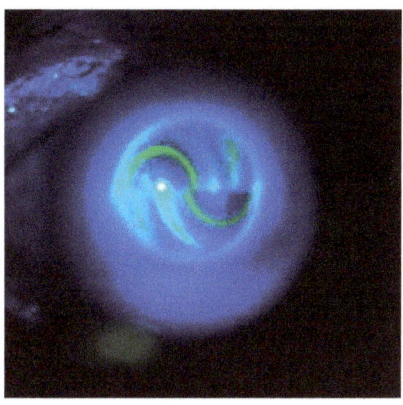

Fig. 3. The end point for eye pressure measurement showing the two semi-circles viewed through the slit-lamp biomicroscope just overlapping.

Because eye pressure was for so long part of the definition of glaucoma and because it is one of the major risk factors to develop glaucoma and the risk factor we modify with our treatment, we need to understand a bit more about it.

Pressure is generated in the eye very simply: there is a circular cellular pump in the eye (the ciliary body) that pushes a clear watery fluid (the aqueous) into the eye from the blood (see Figure 4). This carries essential nutrients like sugars, vitamins and minerals and some protein into the eye to nourish the living structures in the eye that cannot be supplied by blood, like the rest of

Glaucoma: How to Save Your Sight!

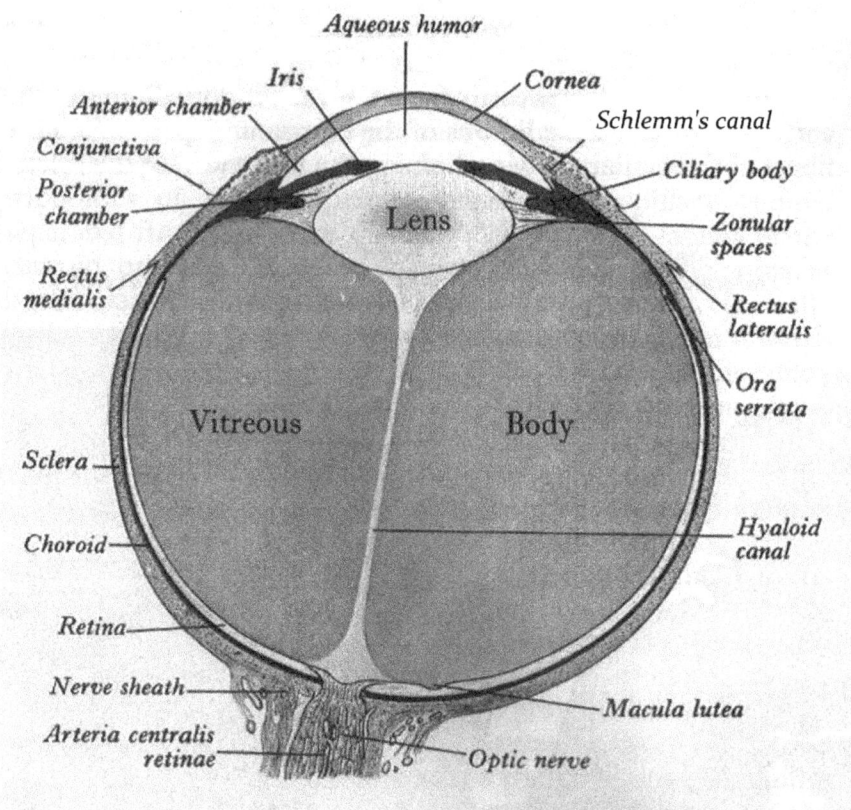

Fig. 4. Schematic diagram of eye ball. From the blood, the ciliary body pumps aqueous into the posterior chamber of the eye. Some of it percolates slowly through the vitreous, but most of it passes between lens and iris, through the pupil, and circulates within the anterior chamber before draining back into the blood-stream. Resistance to outflow creates eye pressure, which is transmitted throughout the eye; it is at the rear, at the beginning of the optic nerve that it damages the exiting nerves carrying the messages of sight.

3. Setting the scene for the seven 'sins'

the body. Why not? Because blood is opaque and these living structures (especially the cornea and the focusing lens) need to be able to transmit light effectively to the nerve network at the back of the eye (the retina, akin to the old fashioned film in a camera).

The aqueous circulates within the eye before draining back to the blood stream through a couple of different pathways, one called conventional, the other, unsurprisingly, unconventional (because it was identified later). While the conventional outflow is through a strainer mesh called the trabeculum into Schlemm's canal and then back to the tiny veins in the front of the eye, the unconventional pathway (also called the uveoscleral pathway) is directly through the eye's internal focusing muscle and then through its wall (the sclera) into the socket in the skull in which the eye lives (the orbit).

As the eye is a closed ball, resistance to aqueous flow in these outflow pathways generates pressure. It is a balance between speed of inflow versus rate of outflow just like the water level in a basin depends on how fast the water flows in through the tap versus how fast it drains out. Because the eye is a closed sphere, any pressing on the eyeball will increase internal pressure, sometimes dramatically.

Pressure in each eye fluctuates all the time; it is known as a *continuous variable*. The environment of the eye is dynamic. Drinking a lot of fluid rapidly increases pump inflow rates and causes swelling of some structures within the eye raising its internal pressure; raising pressure in the veins into which the aqueous empties, increases pressure (coughing, holding one's breath as in straining, playing a wind musical instrument, lying down) increases eye pressure; pressing on the eyeball causes a spike in pressure (finger eye rubbing, small tight swimming goggles, eyelid squeezing, even normal eye blinking momentarily). While the tissues of the eye normally cope with these often wide fluctuations, eyes with glaucoma damage may suffer.

When we measure eye pressure in the clinic situation, we are sampling this continuously varying risk factor. We base our recommendations on a very small part of reality. Until we have ways of measuring pressure accurately and frequently (if not constantly) this is the current state of our possible care.

Damage to the optic nerve might be caused by the level of average pressures, by peaks in pressure that could occur at any time, by the variations in the pressure from minimum to maximum or by some combination of all of these. Assessing how the optic nerve fibres cope with these variations is critically important.

So what does the optic nerve look like when viewed with instruments from the front? We are now discussing the structure of the nerves as they run to the opening at the back of the eye where they turn to exit and as they negotiate that turn and head off towards the brain.

Imagine a single opening in the back of each eye. All the nerve fibres from the retina, carrying the messages of sight, converge towards that opening where they

3. Setting the scene for the seven 'sins'

turn through 90 degrees and exit the eye together, forming the optic nerve. As they cascade out of the eye, the view from the front is like looking down at a huge waterfall (imagine the Niagara Falls) from a helicopter. A dimple forms in the centre where there are no nerve fibres. We call this dimple the 'cup'. It is a bit like a halved avocado where the pip has been removed, leaving a cavity. In glaucoma, this cavity enlarges by default as the nerve fibres are killed and disappear. The surrounding rim of remaining cascading nerve fibres thins and the cavity deepens and widens as the surrounding nerves disappear (Figures 5, 6 & 7).

For diagnosis, the critical signs are a deep, large cup with a thin and perhaps irregular remaining nerve rim. When you have your eye examination, **it is as important to ask your ophthalmologist about your optic nerves as it is to ask about your eye pressure levels.**

Some people, however, inherit a large optic cup while others may have a cup that is small and shallow. This wide variation in the normal population may make it difficult to detect early glaucoma damage, as large cups might be normal for that individual and small cups may disguise early damage.

Optic nerve evaluation is an essential part of the eye examination. When necessary, it should be supplemented by photographs and scanned images from advanced technologies such as scanning laser ophthalmoscopy, scanning laser polarimetry and ocular coherent tomography. These devices have an error rate

Glaucoma: How to Save Your Sight!

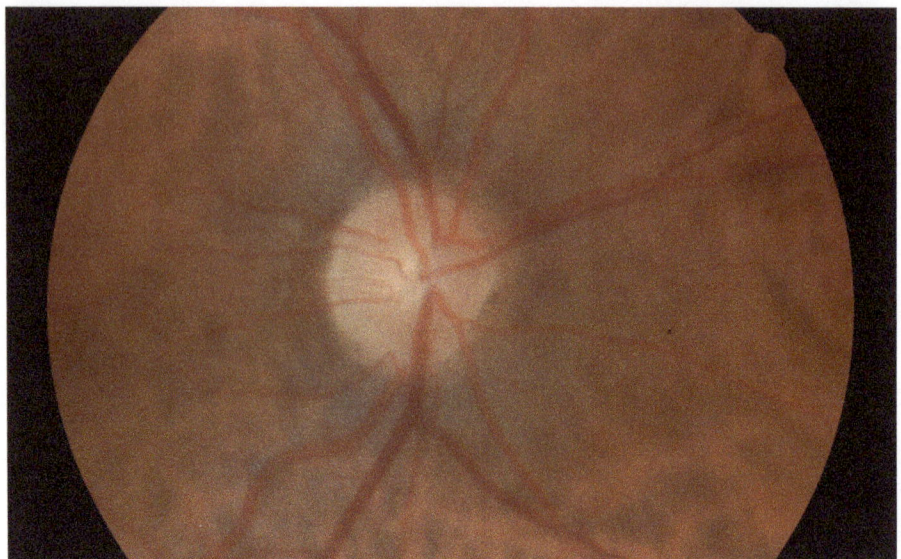

Fig. 5. Right normal optic nerve head (optic disc) seen from the front. In the center we see a normal dimple, called the 'cup'.

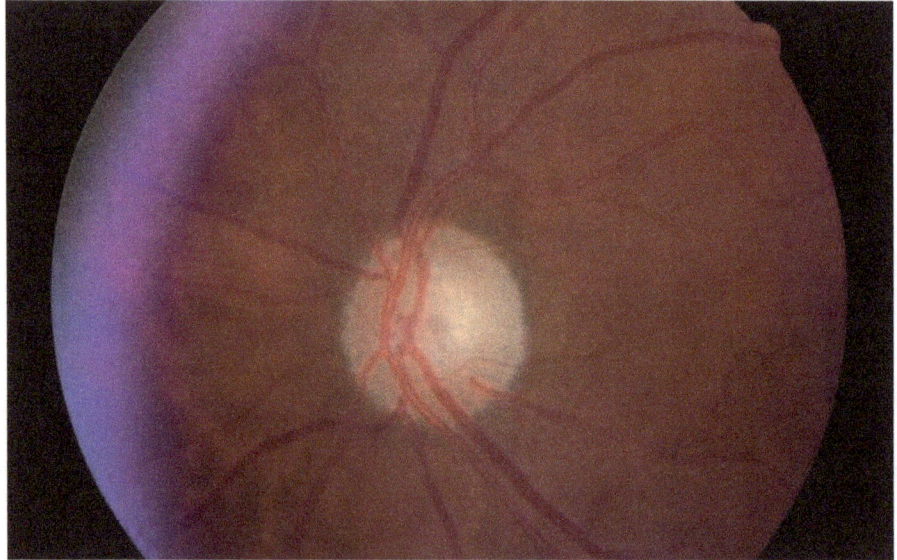

Fig. 6. Left optic disc with moderate glaucoma damage. Note the thinner pink rim, especially in the upper and lower sectors and the vertical extension and widening of the cup.

3. Setting the scene for the seven 'sins'

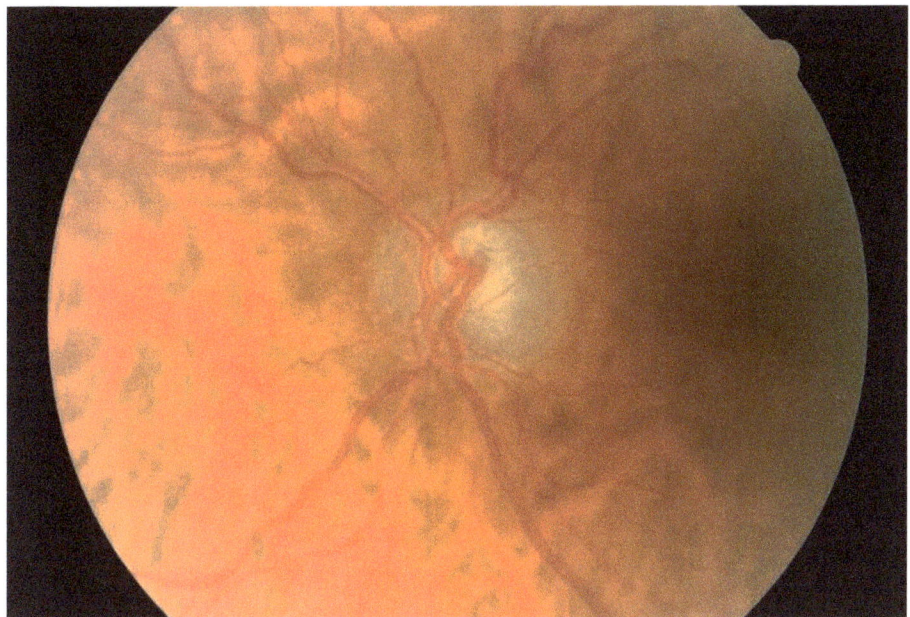

Fig. 7. Left optic disc with advanced damage. See how the rim is paler than before and how very thin it is, again, especially above and below. The blood vessels are no longer supported by the nerve tissues and have fallen outwards to the edges of the opening at the rear of the eye.

of approximately 15% in 'diagnosing' healthy people as having glaucoma and conversely in suggesting glaucoma patients are 'normal'. Diagnosis cannot be based solely on their assessments, but to be as accurate as possible, must be made with mutually supportive information from the entire examination and assessment.

It is not good for healthy people to be treated needlessly, nor for glaucoma patients to be reassured wrongly that they do not need treatment.

As the nerves run to the back of the eye from all over

the retina, carrying the messages of sight, they form thickened bundles, like highways. Glaucoma damage kills these nerve fibres and as they die and disappear, these bundles thin. This can be observed and measured with the same instruments that measure the shape of the nerves as they exit the eye, also known as the optic nerve head (like the head of a river).

All this allows the assessment of nerve structure.

Another, equally important assessment is of nerve performance or function. This is tested by using computers to measure sensitivity of the eye in different locations of sight to light stimulation and is called visual field testing or perimetry. Figure 8 shows a Humphrey perimeter.

Often these computers work by shining a tiny light sequentially in many directions onto the inside surface of a white bowl of which the background brightness is fixed. Your head is placed (comfortably we hope) into the bowl, one eye is covered (no peeking allowed) and with your uncovered eye being tested, you are asked to keep looking steadily at a target. This stabilizes the position of your eye and allows the machine to test different parts of your nerve fibres and retina by shining the light into different parts of the bowl.

At each point tested, the brightness of the projected light is varied so that the machine can measure the dimmest light you are able to see at that point. It is a test of light threshold.

3. Setting the scene for the seven 'sins'

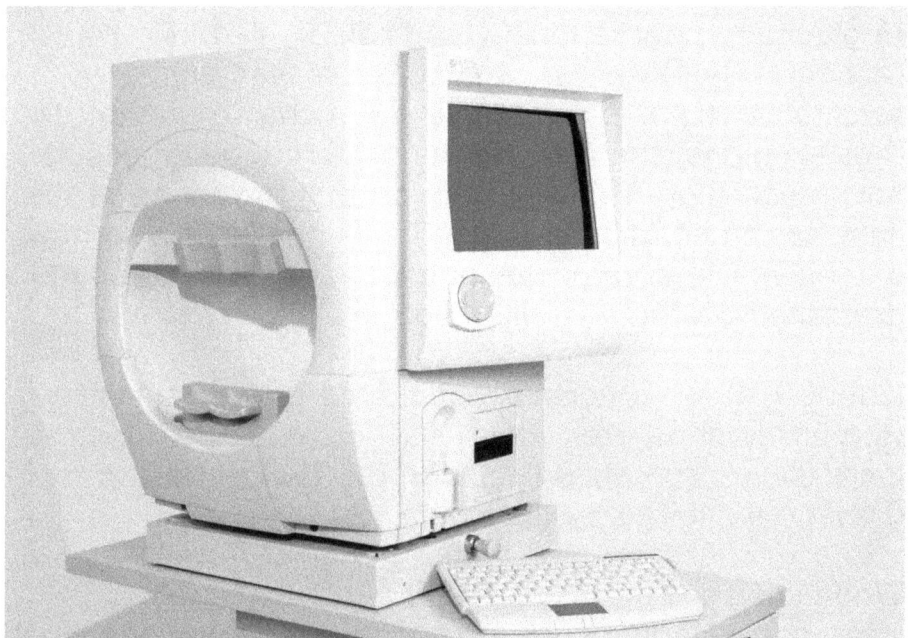

Fig. 8. Humphrey Perimeter

This makes it challenging to do because the light is either just, just bright enough to be seen, or just, just too faint to be seen. You experience doubt and that is perfectly normal. To do the test most effectively, first relax, knowing that about 25% of the time, even in a totally undamaged eye, you will not see the light.

Keep your eye being tested steadily viewing the target and press the button to register you have seen the light *when you think you see it.* Do not wait for it to be a bright flash and do not go looking for it by moving your head or eyes around. See Appendix 2 for tips on how to perform visual field testing to produce an optimal result in the most comfortable way possible.

In glaucoma, nerve fibres tend to be killed in recognizable patterns, causing decreased light sensitivity in parts of the eye like a chain reaction. In those regions, the field machine (perimeter) measures how much more brightly than normal for your age the light has to be for you to see it. It measures also how extensive the area of damage is. Patches of damage are called scotomas ('blind spots').

Figure 9 shows a normal visual field print out from a Humphrey perimeter. Figures 10, 11 & 12 demonstrate increasing visual field loss with the typical patterns of damage exhibited by glaucoma.

When shown their visual field results for the first time, some patients are surprised by the damage that glaucoma has caused: they have not been aware of it. This is because each of us creates a mental model of the world around us, based on the information from the eyes. If bits of information are missing, the brain simply constructs its model on what's available, which might be faulty, sometimes even dangerously so (think of bicycle riding or driving or operating complex machines). Think of the normal situation in which we cannot see behind us, yet our brain constructs a 3-dimensional model for the world around us, including what is behind us, and we move through it without another thought. The same thing happens if part of the visual field has been damaged by glaucoma or by stroke, for example.

Being helped to be aware of the scotoma(s) in each eye can make a big difference to how a patient can

3. Setting the scene for the seven 'sins'

compensate and continue to live a full and productive life safely.

Measuring damage to the visual field is not very sensitive with early glaucoma damage. Up to 50% of the optic nerve fibres may have to be killed before visual fields indicate consistent scotomas. So 'mild' visual field loss may be associated with 'moderate' or even in some cases, severe optic nerve structural damage.

Together with optic nerve structural assessment, visual field loss guides treatment recommendations and allows us to work out whether treatment has halted the disease or whether it is still progressing. If further damage is detected, it usually means treatment has to be made stronger to protect you. Detecting changes in the risk for more damage (higher eye pressure, for example) and assessment for progressive damage is what disease monitoring is all about.

Fig. 9. Normal right single visual field print-out. This is the patient's view of the world. The cross hairs mark the point of fixation, where focused vision is at its peak and where for example, we read, write and recognize faces. The black smudge to the right of fixation highlights the normal ('physiological') blind spot, which is the projection into space of the optic disc itself (it has no photoreceptors and is thus an area in which the eye is totally blind. Besides recording a patient's details, including some of the settings for this test, the print-out indicates how reliably it was performed: false negatives (e.g., a sleepy, tired or distracted subject), false positives (e.g., done with over-zealous, perhaps anxious button-pressing) and fixation losses (someone looking for the light rather than watching the target straight ahead). The software also calculates the significance of any depression in sensitivities at every point tested, correcting for the patient's age, and then highlights this graphically with black squares.

3. Setting the scene for the seven 'sins'

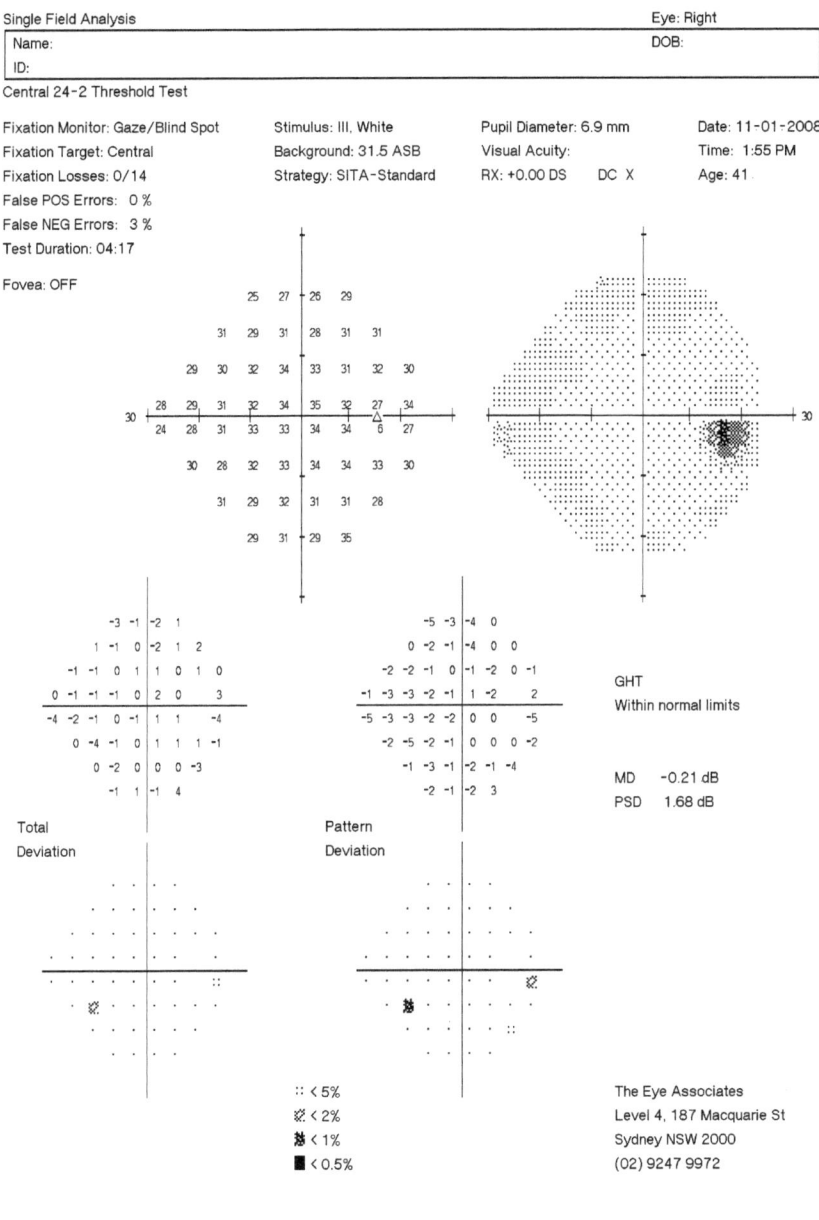

Fig. 10. Early visual field loss from glaucoma. As this is the left eye, note the positioning of the normal blind spot black smudge to the left of the point of fixation. See how the software has highlighted with extra dots and shading a significant drop in light detection sensitivity in a cluster of tested points above and along the horizontal on the nose side of the person's outlook (arrow). As this finding was reproducible and consistent and also importantly matched changes in the optic disc nerve fibre thickness, it shows real, but at this stage early glaucoma vision damage. The patient was completely unaware of this defect in his vision.

3. Setting the scene for the seven 'sins'

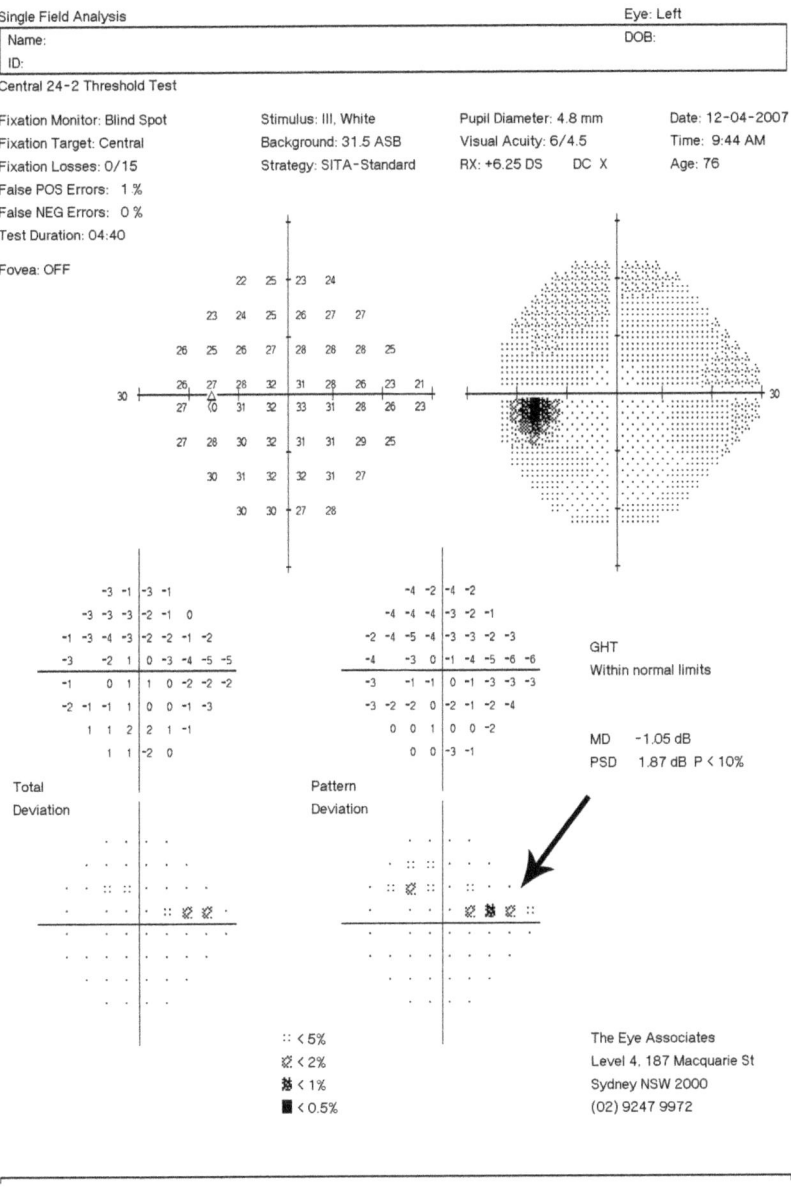

Fig. 11. Moderate visual field loss in a right eye from glaucoma. See how the blind spot (scotoma) is to the right of fixation in this right eye. Here visual damage is moderate: there is an arc of damage highlighted by the software with black squares. This is an example of an inferior (below the horizontal) arcuate (arc-shaped) glaucomatous scotoma. Once again, the patient was totally unaware of this defect until it was pointed out and explained.

3. Setting the scene for the seven 'sins'

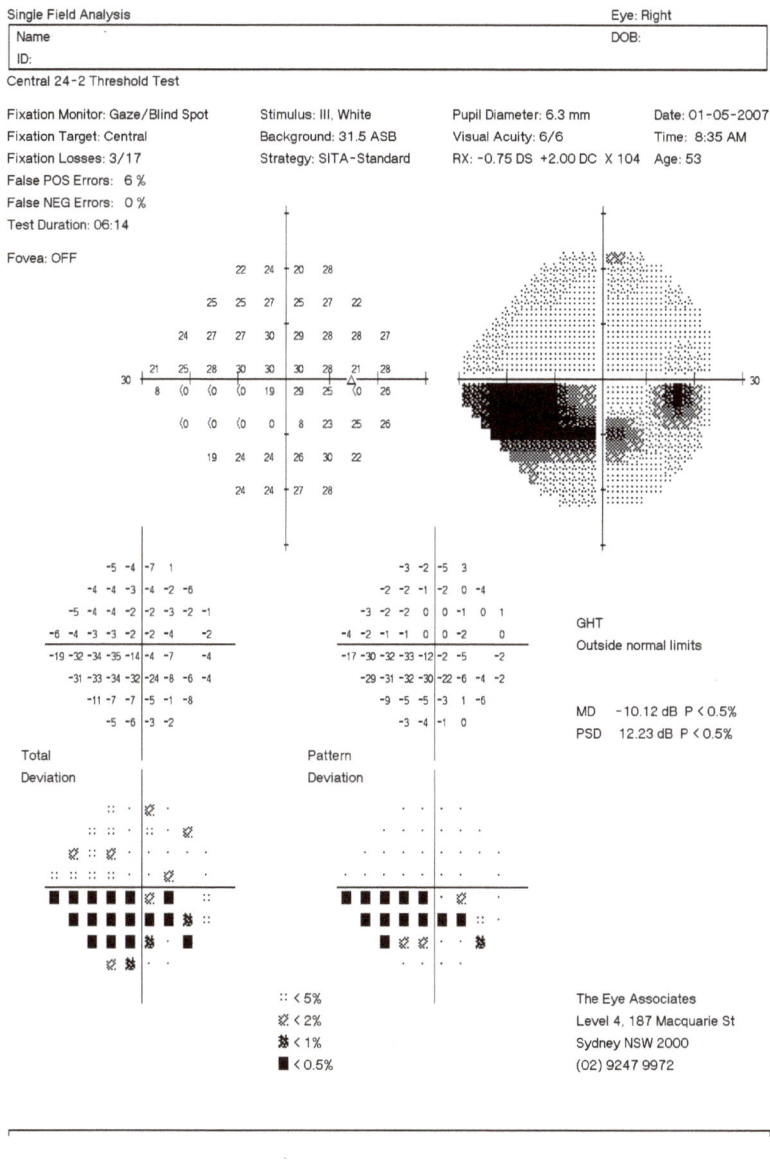

Fig. 12. Extensive ('end-stage') visual field loss from glaucoma in a left eye. The black squares indicate extensive dramatic loss in vision both above and below the horizontal such that the arcuate scotomas have joined together to form a circle. Remaining vision is a central tunnel and a crescent out to the left side. At this stage of loss, most patients are aware of visual disability: their mobility can be restricted, especially if the other eye also has damage and falls or injuries are more common.

3. Setting the scene for the seven 'sins'

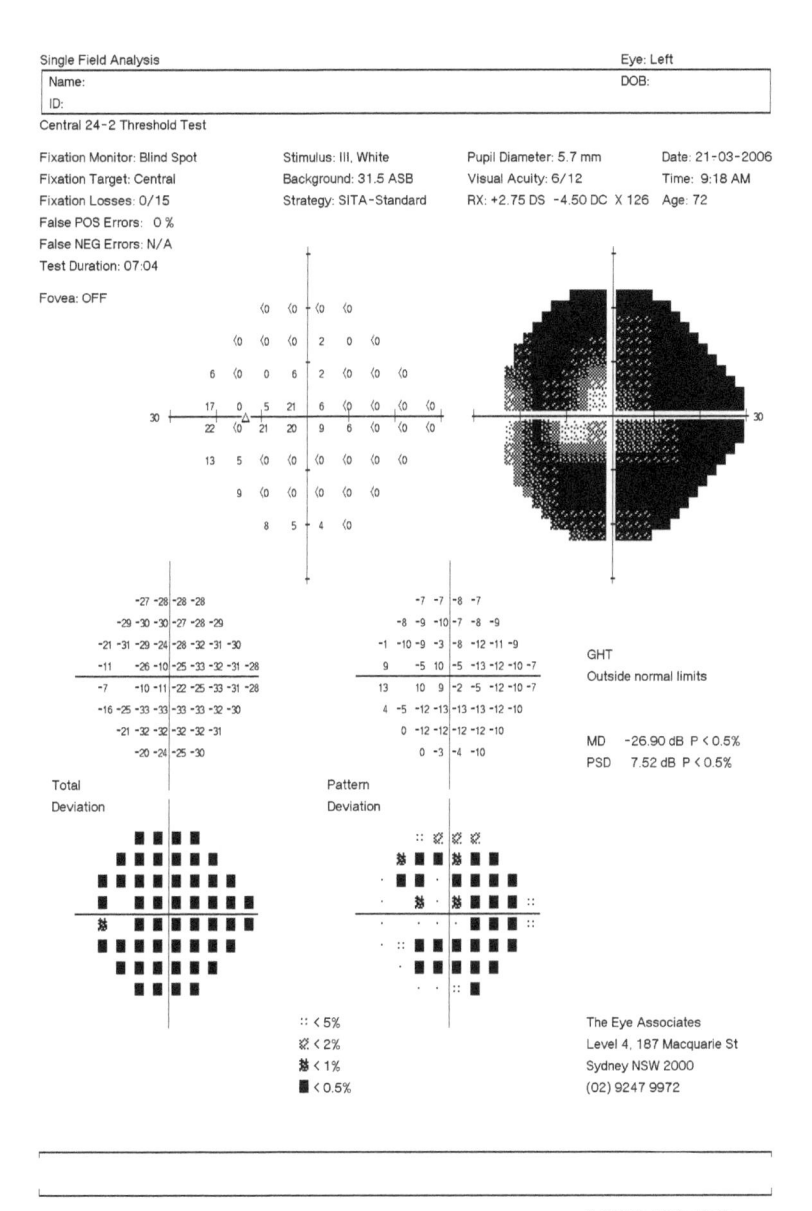

Single Field Analysis	Eye: Left
Name:	DOB:
ID:	

Central 24-2 Threshold Test

Fixation Monitor: Blind Spot   Stimulus: III, White   Pupil Diameter: 5.7 mm   Date: 21-03-2006
Fixation Target: Central   Background: 31.5 ASB   Visual Acuity: 6/12   Time: 9:18 AM
Fixation Losses: 0/15   Strategy: SITA-Standard   RX: +2.75 DS -4.50 DC X 126   Age: 72
False POS Errors: 0 %
False NEG Errors: N/A
Test Duration: 07:04

Fovea: OFF

GHT
Outside normal limits

MD   -26.90 dB   P < 0.5%
PSD   7.52 dB   P < 0.5%

Total Deviation   Pattern Deviation

:: < 5%
※ < 2%
▨ < 1%
■ < 0.5%

The Eye Associates
Level 4, 187 Macquarie St
Sydney NSW 2000
(02) 9247 9972

© 2005 Carl Zeiss Meditec
HFA II 750-10676-4.0/4.0

3.2 Sin 2: Failing to detect progressive damage

If your treatment program is not reviewed at timely intervals or if you fail to attend for follow-up assessments or if you do not undergo some of the additional investigations (such as visual fields or optic disc measurements) as required, you are increasing the chances of failing to detect ongoing damage to your sight.

Glaucoma tends to be relentless. It seizes opportunities to destroy. It has been likened to the ocean: as you never know when the next big wave is going to come through, you never take your eyes off it. You remain vigilant. You remain alert and informed.

You and your ophthalmologist are allies against the disease. Together you need to work out a treatment strategy that is likely to work to make you safe and then to check regularly that you have been made safe.

No glaucoma patient on treatment should go for more than a year between assessments. Most glaucoma patients need three- to six-monthly reviews, depending on the severity of the damage and the apparent stability of the condition from treatment. The milder the damage, the more effective the treatment, the longer the follow-up demonstrating stability, the longer the safe interval between visits. Figure 13 shows an overview of three visual fields with possible progressive damage. Figure 14 shows two visual fields with no apparent change.

3. Setting the scene for the seven 'sins'

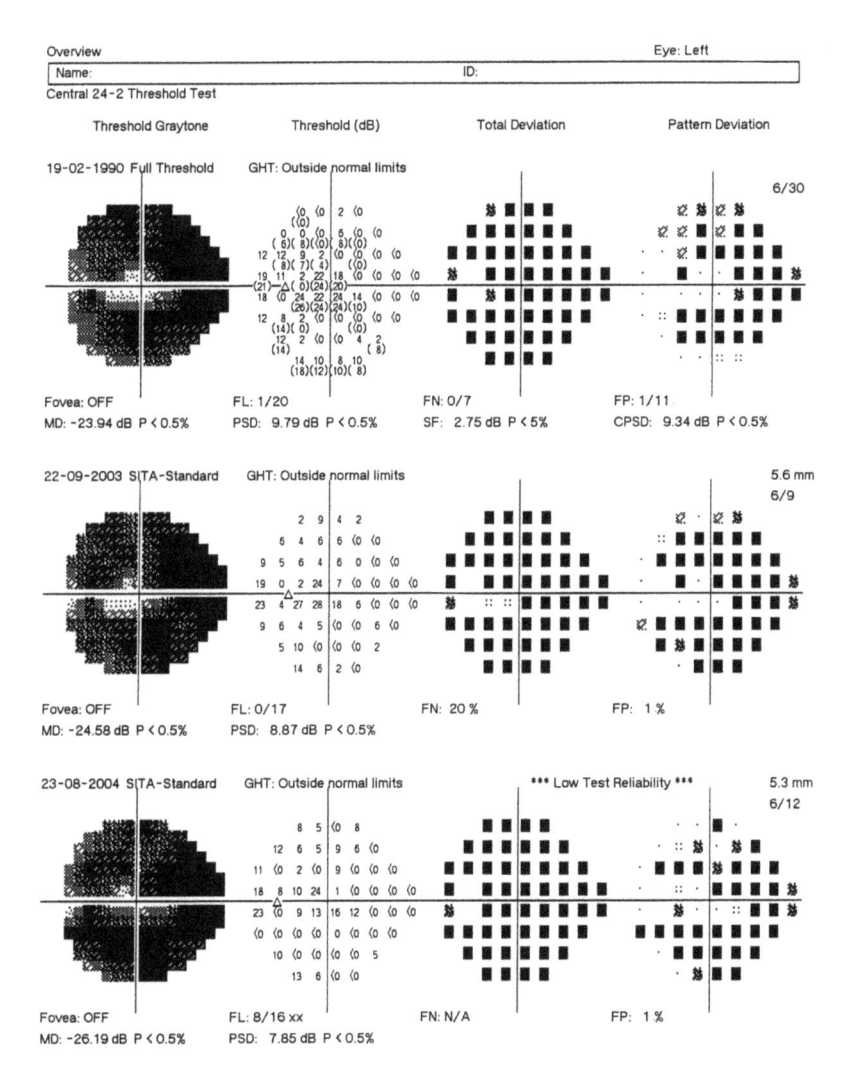

Fig. 13. Overview printout of three left visual fields of an eye with very advanced damage over a 14-year period. Possible progression in damage is shown by an increase in the mean deviation (MD) parameter from -23.94 to -26.19. Interpretation needs to take into account the significant number of fixation losses (FL) and in the past, the rate of false negatives (FN). Performing a ten-degree central visual field would help to understand the stability or instability of the central tunnel of vision.

Fig. 14. Left visual fields showing mild to moderate damage as an inferior arcuate scotoma, which seems unchanged over an eight-month period. The relatively small number of false positive (FP) errors does not affect interpretation.

3. Setting the scene for the seven 'sins'

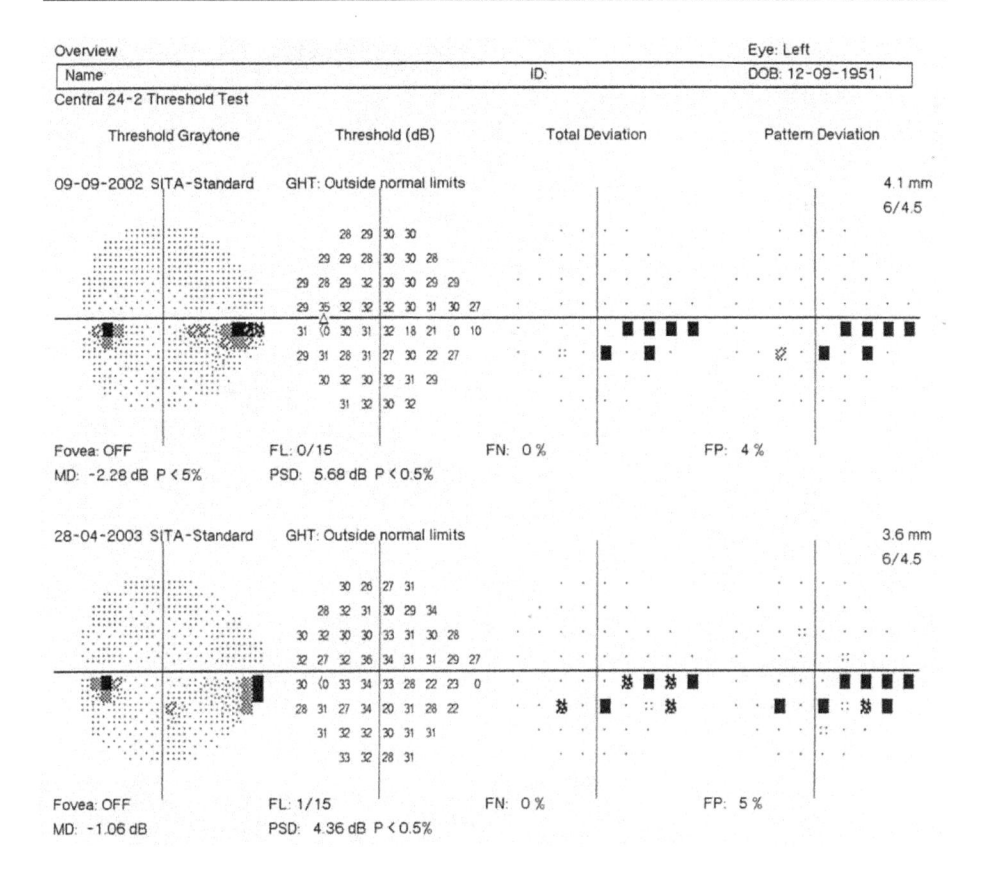

Overview   Eye: Left
Name   ID: DOB: 12-09-1951
Central 24-2 Threshold Test

Threshold Graytone	Threshold (dB)	Total Deviation	Pattern Deviation

09-09-2002 SITA-Standard   GHT: Outside normal limits   4.1 mm
6/4.5

```
              28 29 30 30
           29 29 28 30 30 28
        29 28 29 32 30 30 29 29
        29 35 32 32 32 30 31 30 27
        31 (0 30 31 32 18 21  0 10
        29 31 28 31 27 30 22 27
           30 32 30 32 31 29
              31 32 30 32
```

Fovea: OFF   FL: 0/15   FN: 0 %   FP: 4 %
MD: -2.28 dB P < 5%   PSD: 5.68 dB P < 0.5%

28-04-2003 SITA-Standard   GHT: Outside normal limits   3.6 mm
6/4.5

```
              30 26 27 31
           28 32 31 30 29 34
        30 32 30 30 33 31 30 28
        32 27 32 36 34 31 31 29 27
        30 (0 33 34 33 28 22 23  0
        28 31 27 34 20 31 28 22
           31 32 32 30 31 31
              33 32 28 31
```

Fovea: OFF   FL: 1/15   FN: 0 %   FP: 5 %
MD: -1.06 dB   PSD: 4.36 dB P < 0.5%

3.3 Sin 3: Failure to differentiate between glaucoma sub-types

Effective treatment depends on an accurate diagnosis and this is entirely the ophthalmologist's responsibility. There must be a separation between open angle, angle closure and secondary glaucomas for each person and you should understand what kind of glaucoma you have. An important part of the eye examination to help to achieve this is gonioscopy. Figure 15 captures the appearance of the anterior chamber angle showing the trabecular meshwork. Figure 16 is a cartoon of the same structures.

Most glaucomas are called *primary*. This means they occur without any detectable cause. Secondary glaucomas occur in eyes with a condition that leads to

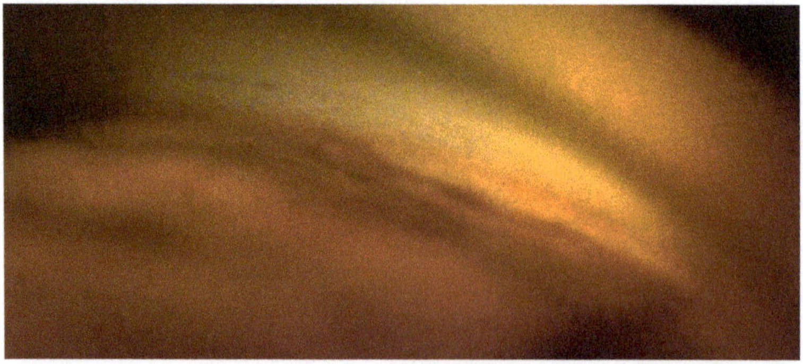

Fig. 15. Slit-lamp view through a gonioscope showing the inside of the cornea above, the coloured iris below and between the two the band of the trabecular meshwork drain. See how to the left side of the photo the iris is caught forwards against the drain by scar tissue called peripheral anterior synechiae caused by scarring that follows prolonged repeated knocking of the meshwork by the iris.

3. Setting the scene for the seven 'sins'

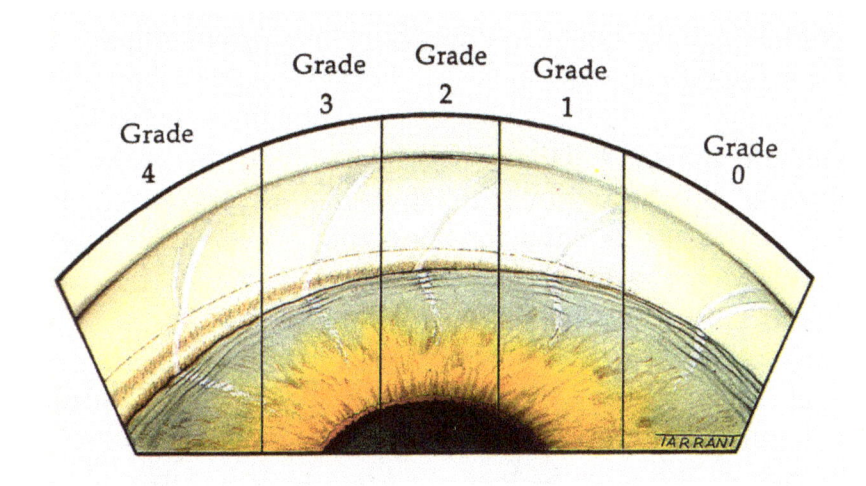

Fig. 16. Schematic drawing of gonioscopic view of the drainage angle showing progressive narrowing from left to right. To the left, the drainage angle is wide open and the trabecular meshwork is totally unobstructed. To the right, as the iris totally blocks the meshwork, the angle is closed.

the problem, such as previous injuries, prolonged use of medications called steroids, inflammation in the eye (iritis or uveitis) or problems with the focusing lens or cornea (the front window or watch-glass of the eye).

One example of a secondary glaucoma is pigmentary glaucoma, which tends to affect slightly short-sighted men in their 20s and 30s. Pigment granules from the back of the iris are dislodged by rubbing, float with the aqueous and become wedged in the trabecular meshwork. Over time, the meshwork's coping mechanisms are overwhelmed, the resistance to outflow increases and the eye pressure rises, putting the optic nerve fibres (and thus the vision) at risk.

The *primary* glaucomas are divided into *open-angle* and *angle-closure* types.

What is the angle? It is the cul-de-sac of the front chamber of the eye known as the anterior chamber, and is made up of the cornea in front and the iris (coloured part of the eye) behind. In the angle is located the conventional outflow pathway for aqueous fluid, the trabecular meshwork. Imagine the thin strip water drain at the bottom of a driveway; take that strip and roll it into a circle and that is what the 0.5-mm wide meshwork is like in your eye, located at the outer circular edge of the coloured part of your eye when you view it from the front.

To access the meshwork and to drain from the eye, the aqueous has to pass along the increasingly narrow space between the cornea and the iris (Figures 1 & 4). Some eyes are built with a deep anterior chamber with a wide open angle, while others are much shallower with a narrow angle. This is entirely the result of what you have inherited from your parents.

As we go through life, the focusing lens behind the iris grows like a tree trunk, gradually expanding over the decades, pushing the iris forwards, shallowing the anterior chamber and narrowing the approaches to the meshwork, *i.e.*, the angle narrows progressively as the decades pass. This is normal and happens to everybody. If you start out with a deep anterior chamber, this does not impact the way the aqueous flows. However, if you start out with a shallow anterior chamber, this progressive narrowing may result in the outer part of

3. Setting the scene for the seven 'sins'

the iris starting to make contact with the meshwork, blocking aqueous outflow, damaging the meshwork and causing the eye pressure to rise.

Gonioscopy identifies this situation. As the treatment for these situations is different from approaches to open-angle glaucomas, it must be identified as early in the treatment process as possible. There are several kinds of medicines, for different conditions, taken orally that are not wise in someone with angle-closure glaucoma, especially if they have not had a laser treatment to try to rectify this (see page 109).

Always ask your ophthalmologist what kind of glaucoma you have and ensure you understand the approaches to treatment that is necessary for you specifically.

3.4 Sin 4: Improperly staging disease severity

Patients with life-threatening conditions often are admitted to intensive-care wards, while those with mild to moderate diseases may be treated in hospital wards or the outpatients department. The same principles apply in glaucoma management – without the threat to life.

A glaucoma patient might have a normal conventional (white light projected onto a white surface) visual field, suggesting early disease and no need for intensive therapy. However, more selective perimetry, with frequency-doubling or ring technologies for example, might reveal extensive areas of visual field impairment. Optic disc imaging may demonstrate severe retinal nerve fibre loss.

Such a difference between conventional and alternative perimetric techniques might occur because of the preponderance of various types of retinal cells. Whereas conventional perimetry tests all cells and results are dominated by the responses of the more common parvo-cellular (small cells) group, alternative perimetry might test selectively the less common magno-cells (large cells). With fewer magno-cells to start with, the glaucoma-induced loss of a smaller number of them might be evident more quickly. The larger number of parvo-cells means there is more redundancy (reserve or 'slack') in those parts of the visual system and therefore more damage is necessary before the tests can detect loss.

3. Setting the scene for the seven 'sins'

This is one way in which glaucoma might be 'sneaky'. While the ophthalmologist watches for damage onset or progression with standard perimetry (achromatic or 'white target light on a white background'), many cells might be destroyed 'silently'.

Non-recognition of this process could result in treatment being inadequate and in failure to accelerate it in the face of disease progression. Because the gap between IOP levels where damage occurred and the IOP levels from treatment is the margin for visual safety, the more severe the damage, the lower the IOP needs to be made to protect against further damage. Sometimes surgery is needed to achieve a sufficiently low IOP.

To add to these technology-related limitations facing the ophthalmologist, unawareness of the severity of the condition by the patient might lead to non-adherence and non-persistence with therapy.

3.5 Sin 5: Insufficient reduction in the eye pressure

In a large Swedish study, 45% of treated patients with an average 25% IOP reduction (about 5 mmHg from untreated baseline) continued to show disease progression. For them, this amount of IOP lowering was insufficient for visual safety. **Each patient needs enough IOP reduction to reach a safe level, determined by the ophthalmologist as his/her 'target' IOP.**

Determining what is the 'target' IOP for a patient is a calculated guess by the ophthalmologist depending on disease severity, life expectancy, the untreated or unsafe IOP levels, the closeness of measured vision damage to the point of fixation (which we use to read, write, recognize faces, watch TV, use computers, for example) and the presence of other contributory conditions such as central corneal thickness.

From several large prospective clinical studies, it seems a 30% IOP reduction should prove sufficient to safeguard vision in the majority of patients with mild to moderate glaucoma. For those with more advanced damage, sometimes a 40 to 50% reduction is required. Often this translates to an absolute IOP of 18 mmHg or less for mild disease, of 15 mmHg or less for moderate damage and for 12 mmHg or less for those with advanced loss.

While the concept of target IOP is helpful to guide treatment strategies, it must be flexible for each

3. Setting the scene for the seven 'sins'

patient: what might be safe when the patient is in his/her 50s, might not be safe in the same patient when he/she is in the 60s. Other conditions, such as high blood pressure being treated simultaneously, onset of diabetes, or sleep apnoea, for example, could all require a change in IOP targets. Even though the ophthalmologist is not treating the whole patient, he/she takes into the account the health of the whole person in order to treat the eyes properly.

Once a target IOP has been estimated and treatment adjusted to achieve it, to be effective, ongoing care demands monitoring to ensure the IOP is indeed safe for that patient at that time. This is 'intelligent use of time'.

Like blood pressure, eye pressures fluctuate second to second (with the heartbeat, for example, playing a wind musical instrument or eye ball movements), from hour to hour (depending on fluid intake, exercise or daily rhythms in hormone levels), from day to day and from season to season (higher in winter, lower in summer). Measuring it just once every few months only gives a hint at its level. Daily peaks in IOP might be as important in glaucoma damage as daily averages. However, to measure the IOP every few hours is not practical and the various self-use home tonometers have not proved reliable, accurate or reproducible in most patients' experience.

One way shown to help reveal peak daily pressures is the water drinking challenge test (WDT).

After a couple of hours of liquid fasting, a patient either drinks 800 ml of water or 10 ml of water for each kilogram of body weight. IOP is measured before and at 15, 30, 45 and sometimes 60 minutes after drinking. IOP increases to a peak and then starts to fall. In about 87% of patients, the peak IOP after the WDT corresponds closely to the peak daily IOP. If the peak detected on treatment is above target levels for that patient, perhaps treatment should be changed so as not only to reduce IOP, but to blunt its peak levels as well.

The WDT resembles cardiac stress tests with exercise, which are widely used by cardiologists. The concept of stress tests is well known outside the field of ophthalmology.

3.6 Sin 6: Delayed early treatment

Based on studies with small populations and relatively short follow-up periods, a decade ago a group of internationally renowned glaucoma sub-specialists argued that early-stage glaucoma might not require treatment. Treatment should be instituted early, they urged only in glaucomas secondary to some other eye conditions, those with high eye pressures and in young people (as with their long life expectancy, there was a greater risk of visual disability). These situations are less common and if this opinion prevailed, the overwhelming majority of glaucoma patients might not receive treatment until their disease had caused moderate damage, or worse.

This same group of colleagues recommended not treating those patients whose rate of visual damage would be unlikely to affect their quality of life, taking into account their anticipated life expectancy.

Such a passive and almost nihilistic clinical approach we view with alarm. **No clinician is able to foresee with certainty how long an individual patient is likely to live, nor how rapidly the condition may progress in future years.** Although software programs that interpret visual field results have improved greatly and can predict likely progression for the next five years based on progression of damage over the past several years, they are not a fool-proof method to guide treatment strategies if used exclusively. It is too easy to place excessive reliance on their accuracy.

Fortunately, these colleagues appreciated the dangers inherent in their advice and these non-treatment concepts now have been consigned to history.

3.7 Sin 7: Patient non-adherence to treatment recommendations

Non-adherence is the accidental or purposeful failure to follow a doctor's direct or implied recommended treatments. It is sometimes known as non-compliance. Another aspect of non-adherence is failure to persist

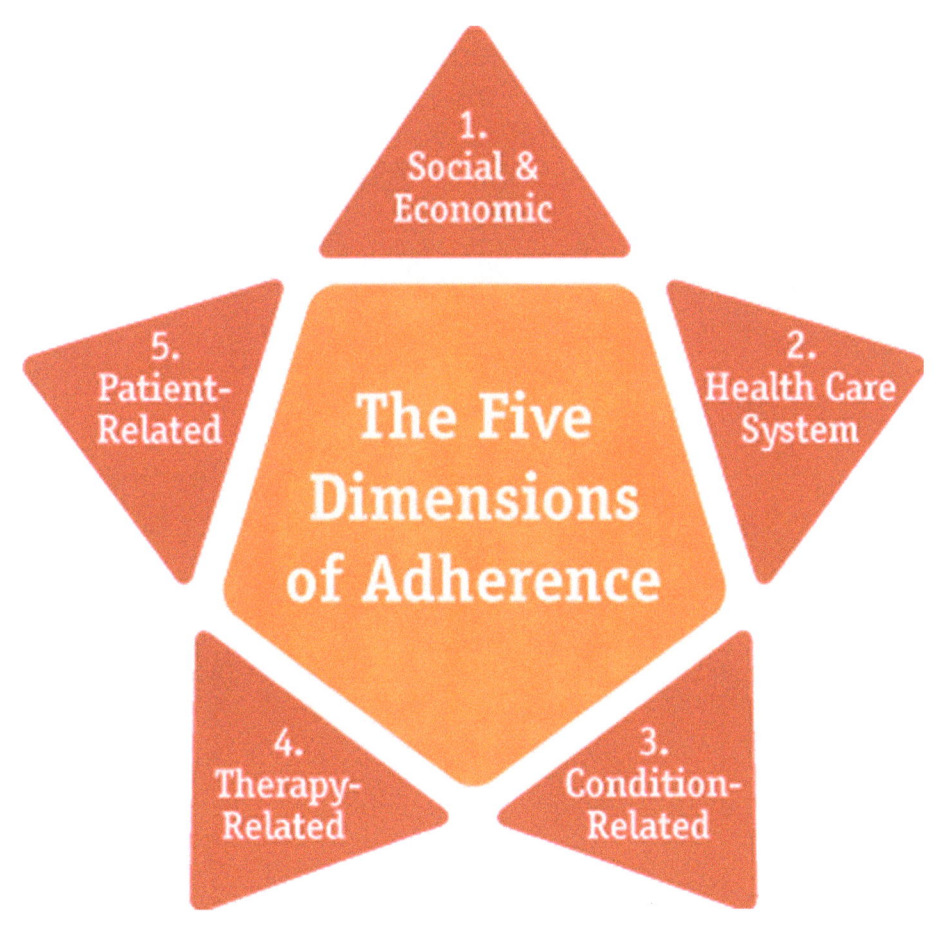

Fig. 17. Five broad dimensions that alone or in combination influence an individual's adherence. (World Health Organisation, 2003)

with a treatment program over time. Yet another encompasses the physical barriers to self-administration of a medication - this applies particularly to the ability to instil eye drops.

Multiple factors affect an individual's adherence; it seems to be a combination of these factors that determines adherence. The World Health Organisation has outlined five broad dimensions or factors, which may affect adherence (Figure 17). The combination relevant for any individual may well change over time. Possible reasons are set out in Figure 18.

Why are Glaucoma Patients Non-Adherent?

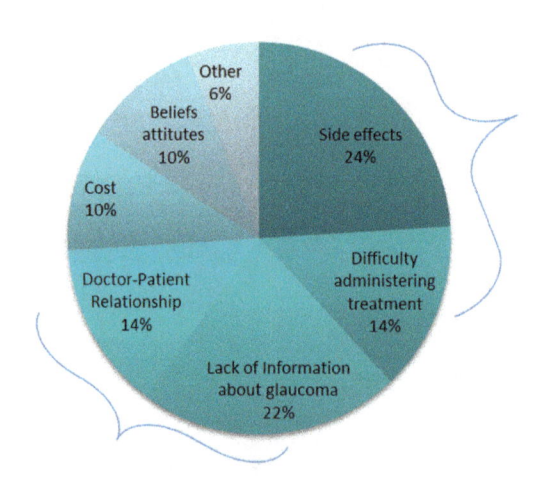

- Other 6%
- Beliefs attitutes 10%
- Side effects 24%
- Cost 10%
- Difficulty administering treatment 14%
- Doctor-Patient Relationship 14%
- Lack of Information about glaucoma 22%

Fig. 18. Reasons within the five broad dimensions for non-adherence in glaucoma patients.

3. Setting the scene for the seven 'sins'

Non-adherence can occur at any time during management, from failure to initiate treatment, through reliable initiation but then abandonment, to improper use of medications in an ongoing and/or erratic manner (Figure 19).

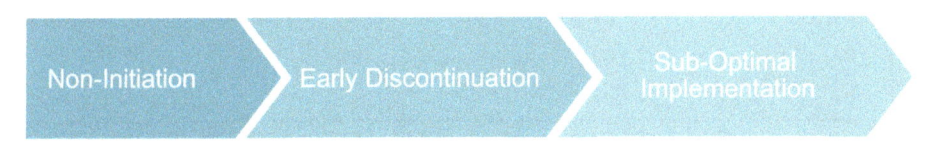

Non-Initiation → Early Discontinuation → Sub-Optimal Implementation

Fig. 19. Various stages of management in which non-adherence might occur.

There are real consequences that may flow from non-adherence (Figure 20).

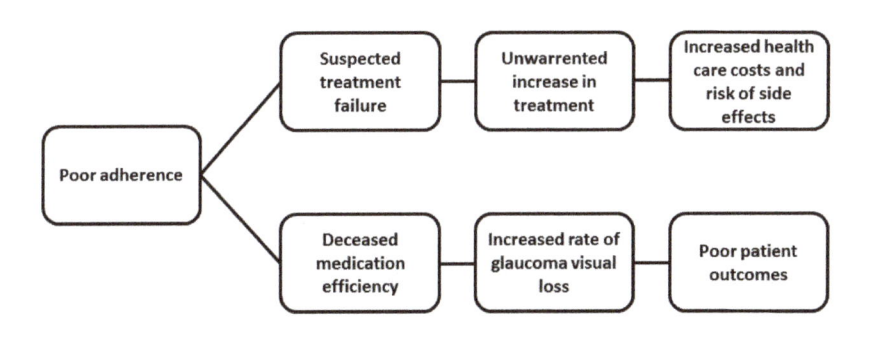

Fig. 20. If drops are used just before a visit but not between visits, visual damage may be worse but IOP seems 'controlled' during that consultation. The ophthalmologist may increase treatment (unnecessarily as the original treatment is working but not being used) with additional drugs to try to lower IOP further with an increased risk of side effects, increased costs and increased complexity of therapy.

The more eye drops needed each day, the less a person tends to adhere. In one study, for example, the following percentages of patients failed in one way or another:

Prescribed	Adherence to the advice	Instillation at correct times
1x	79%	74%
2x	69%	58%
3x	65%	46%
4x	51%	40%

Some patients deliberately cease their eye drops before their regular visit to the ophthalmologist to see if they 'really' need to keep using them. If their eye pressure happens to fall into the 'normal' range, they wrongly assume the medicine isn't necessary. It shows complete misunderstanding of the sinister nature of glaucoma.

Some patients forget or avoid their eye drops between visits, but remember to use them when they are coming in to see their ophthalmologist. After the visit, particularly if no further damage

3. Setting the scene for the seven 'sins'

has been detected, they continue to use their medicines erratically.

This is like leaving the front door of your home unlocked. If a thief does not try the lock, you would not lose anything. However, if a thief happens to test the door and finds easy access, you might or might not notice that you've been robbed. It is the same with glaucoma and your sight: you might get away with it (for a time) or you might lose some vision, but not notice, or you might lose some vision that you notice immediately (especially if it is close to the centre of your sight, which you need to read, write, watch TV, recognize faces and so on).

Your vision is like a piece of cheese: there is a certain amount of it and no more. Glaucoma is like a mouse nibbling away at the cheese: what's eaten is gone forever, it cannot be regained. Our treatment can paralyse the mouse, but cannot kill it – **we can slow or halt the glaucoma, but we cannot cure it.** Keeping the eye pressure down is what makes your vision safe, by stopping the disease process. If the treatment is used erratically and the pressures fluctuate, the disease claims a little more and then a little more of your non-renewable vision, just as the mobile mouse is able to swallow a little more of the cheese.

Follow the treatment plan you have worked out for you with your ophthalmologist. If you find you are not able to do so, for any reason, be sure to discuss it with him or her. Lowering your eye pressure to make your vision safe does not need to be done only with eye drops:

there are other possible strategies, like laser techniques and surgery. So if one program doesn't work for you, admit it to yourself and tell your ophthalmologist. Then you will be able to work out an alternative program that will make your sight safe.

Remember, your ophthalmologist is on your side; it is the glaucoma that is the enemy. With your ophthalmologist as your ally against the disease that is attacking you, you should be able to find a solution that works for you.

3. Setting the scene for the seven 'sins'

Focal Points

- Drops don't have to be used at exactly the same time each day: that would be impossible. Try to link them with landmarks in your day, such as after waking, when shaving, with breakfast or dinner, when brushing teeth or when retiring to bed.

- If drops do not reduce your IOP as needed, there are other options such as laser therapy and a variety of incisional surgical procedures.

- In some situations, your doctor may recommend surgical procedures early in your treatment, such as with far advanced glaucoma or a closed drainage system, especially if your eye pressures are very high

- Trabeculectomy remains the "golden standard" among glaucoma surgeries . Your vision is likely to be blurred and to fluctuate after surgery, maybe even for some months. Your ophthalmologist will guide you through this carefully.

- If you've had a glaucoma operation and you develop an infection, seek help immediately.

- Clues that you might have an infection include an eye that is red and irritable, especially with a yellowy pus discharge or with eyelid stickiness, particularly when you awake in the mornings.

4. Glaucoma treatment

What is known to make vision safe is reduction in both peak and average eye pressure: in fact the gap between eye pressure levels when damage was occurring and eye pressures on treatment is the person's visual safety margin.

Even though there are more people with raised eye pressure who do not have glaucoma than people with raised eye pressure who *do* have glaucoma and despite the finding that a substantial proportion of glaucoma sufferers have so-called 'normal' eye pressures (30% in Australia, 80% in Korea, 90% in Japan), eye pressure helps to determine risk of onset of glaucoma damage and the risk of that damage progressing.

Traditionally, the glaucoma treatment approach has been to start therapy with single medications in the form of eye drops and if necessary to increase effectiveness by adding additional medicines. If a combination of eye drops cannot be found that is tolerated, not too inconvenient to use and strong enough to lower eye pressures to levels thought to be safe, laser treatment becomes an option: in open-angle glaucoma this is *trabeculoplasty* (a non-incisional surgical technique). Sometimes laser trabeculoplasty may be offered instead of a medication or instead of additional medications. If none of this leads to target eye pressures, incisional surgery is the next step.

In some instances, depending on a number of factors (if eye pressures are very high and damage is advanced, for example), it is possible incisional surgery will be recommended as a very early option. It is the most efficient way to avoid glaucoma progression. However, as incisional surgery might be unpredictable in its results and carries some significant risks to vision (bleeding, infection, cataract formation, for example) it is usually reserved for a later stage in the treatment approach for most patients.

4. Glaucoma treatment

4.1 Treatment with medications (eye drops)

There are five families of medicines that lower eye pressure. To understand how they work, imagine a water basin: water flows from the tap into the basin, it circulates around inside the basin and then runs down the drain. Anything that interferes with the circulation of the water in the basin or the speed with which the fluid is able to pass through the drain will cause the water level in the basin to rise. Similarly, pressure in the eye increases if anything blocks circulation or slows down the drain function.

In concept, the eye is similar: the aqueous is pumped actively into the eye (by the ciliary body), carrying the essential nutrients to the living tissues within. It circulates around inside the eye nourishing the various structures that focus light and then it is removed through one of two outflow pathways. One, the *conventional pathway*, is through a meshwork called the trabeculum; the other is the *unconventional* or *uveo-scleral pathway*. Either way, the fluid returns to the blood stream eventually, to be renewed.

If the circulation within the eye is disturbed, the aqueous fluid cannot reach either drainage system and this is usually caused by one of the *secondary glaucomas* (the result of some other disease process affecting the inside structures of the eye) or *angle closure* (which is caused by steady growth over time of the focusing lens of the eye with progressive crowding of structures when the eye is built in a particular way genetically). As these kinds of blockages can cause eye pressures to rise to very high levels very quickly (like a plug being placed in the water basin's drain), sometimes these different sorts of glaucomas need their own specific treatment programs.

The commonest type, *open-angle glaucoma* has no obvious blockage to the flow of fluid within the eye and no apparent interference with the fluid reaching the drainage pathways. However, those pathways simply do not work fast enough. It is like the drain of the water basin being clogged with tea leaves or some other debris.

So, how do the five families of eye medicines work to reduce eye pressure?

Some of them slow down the rate at which the aqueous fluid is pumped into the eye while others improve the performance of either or both the conventional and unconventional outflow pathways. Combinations of drugs that work by different mechanisms can prove very useful to bring eye pressures down further, if one medicine is not effective enough. In this case, one medicine might slow down the pump while the other might improve outflow drainage, like turning down the tap and cleaning out the drain of the water basin at the same time.

Usually there is one medicine in each bottle of eye drops. Increasingly, fixed combinations of drugs are becoming available around the world. In these, two (or sometimes even more) drugs are placed in the same

4. Glaucoma treatment

bottle, so one drop from one bottle administers two or more medicines. This improves convenience enormously for the patient, it means there is less contact with preservatives in most bottles (to sterilize them, but they can cause irritation to the eye surface), fewer bottles to have to buy each month (saving money) and no need to have to wait at least five minutes between different bottles to improve penetration and thus power of each medicine.

What are the five families? Drugs that reduce the rate of inflow are from the families of beta-blockers, alpha-2 adrenergics and carbonic anhydrase inhibitors.

Beta-Blockers include timolol, bunolol, betaxolol and carteolol. Most widely used is timolol; it became available in 1978 and because it is generally so well-tolerated and effective, it revolutionized medical treatment at that time. Initially it was used routinely twice daily (as the other beta-blockers still are), but later research suggested that for 90% of patients, timolol instilled once daily was just as powerful as used twice daily. Therefore, when prescribed as a single agent or in combination with a prostaglandin analogue, nowadays timolol is often instilled just once daily.

Very rapidly, the majority of use of timolol has become incorporated with another drug into a fixed-combination product. The frequency with which it needs to be used becomes governed by the frequency the companion drug requires. Hence, when combined with a prostaglandin such as latanoprost (XalaCom), travoprost (DuoTrav) or bimatoprost (GanFort), it is recommended just once daily. When combined with a carbonic anhydrase inhibitor such as dorzolamide (Cosopt) or brinzolamide (Azarga) or with an alpha-2 agonist such as brimonindine (Combigan) it is recommended twice daily.

In an appreciable number of patients, timolol may cause potentially serious side effects. It may precipitate or aggravate wheezing, asthma and coughing as well as reduce blood pressure and slow down the heart rate. It must be used cautiously therefore in anyone with breathing or heart problems. Timolol may also mask the warning signs for low blood sugar in patients with insulin-dependent diabetes mellitus (tremor and sweating). All doctors looking after you need to know what eye drops you are using, especially timolol, because of the possible effects on general health.

So-called relatively selective beta-blockers, such as betaxolol (Betoptic) have much less chance of causing breathing or circulation problems than timolol, but may not lower eye pressure as effectively.

Timolol has been described in some patients as contributing to a general feeling of tiredness and lack of energy, to depression, to decreased libido and even to increased hair loss in men. Fortunately, these side effects are relatively uncommon.

One way shown to be effective to decrease general absorption into the body of any drug instilled into the eye and thereby to decrease significantly the chances of any general side effects is to close your eyes without blinking AND to press the pulp of each index finger over

4. Glaucoma treatment

the tear ducts on the nose side of the eyelids for at least two and preferably three minutes after every drop instillation. See Figure 21 and ask your ophthalmologist to show you how it should be done. Blocking the tear ducts retains the medicine in the eye for longer, allowing better penetration and improved effectiveness and at the same time reduces by two-thirds the amount of drug that gets absorbed into your system.

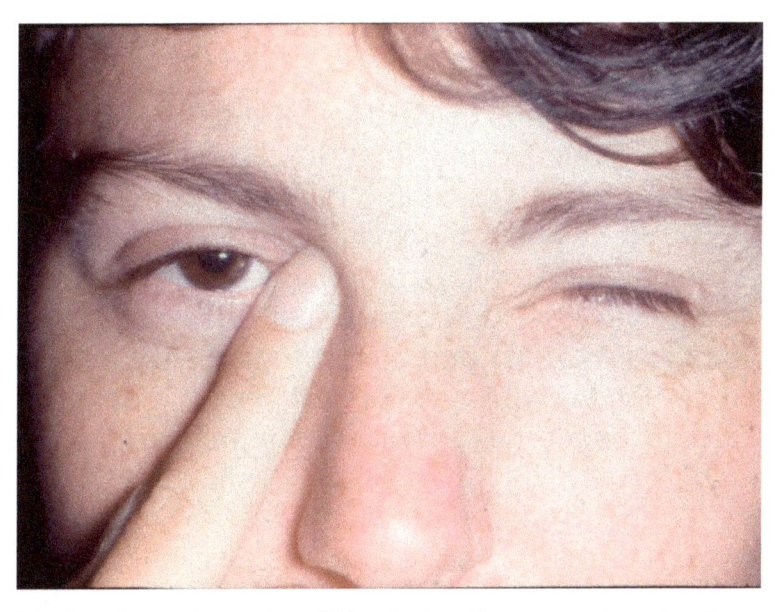

Fig. 21. See how the pulp of the index finger pushes backwards at the nose side of the eyelids (Digital Occlusion of the Tear ducts) and how the left eye is simply closed without blinking (Don't Open Technique). Doing both simultaneously for at least two minutes makes for "double DOT".

Carbonic anhydrase inhibitors have been used to help control IOP since 1954, but for most of that time only as tablets: acetazolamide (Diamox) and methazolamide (Neptazane). They are powerful, but cause significant side effects like lethargy, drowsiness, tingling in the hands and feet, altered taste especially for fizzy drinks, loss of appetite, stomach upsets, muscle cramps and even kidney stones. As they are distantly related to sulpha drugs, anyone allergic to sulpha antibiotics needs to be careful using a carbonic anhydrase inhibitor. Taking tablets with food may help prevent many of these side effects. Because of all this, these tablets are not used often and preferably not for the long-term.

Eye drop preparations of carbonic anhydrase inhibitors only became available in the 1990s. They are not as effective as their tablet sibling drugs, but are much better tolerated. They might cause some eye surface burning for a short while, some redness and a sour taste in the mouth. The commonest ones available are dorzolamide (Trusopt) and brinzolamide (Azopt). These may be combined with timolol and called 'Cosopt' or 'Azarga' respectively; twice daily instillations are necessary.

The alpha-2 adrenergic agonists also became available in the 1990s. While their main effect is to slow down the aqueous pump and thus lower eye pressure, they also might improve unconventional outflow and thus have a dual mechanism of action. These drugs can lower IOP very rapidly, making them useful if there are pressure spikes for any reason. Two are used, twice daily: apraclonidine (Iopidine) and brimonidine (Alphagan, Alphagan-P and Alphagan Z) as stand-alone products, or brimonidine combined with timolol as Combigan. Brimonidine is now also available as a fixed

4. Glaucoma treatment

combination with brinzolamide ("Simbrinza"), which does not contain a beta-blocker.

While the alpha-2 agonists can cause eye redness, itching, dryness, burning and foreign-body sensation, their major handicaps are that the eye often develops resistance (known as tachyphylaxis) especially to apraclonidine and/or an allergic reaction, which may affect up to 25% of patients using brimonidine for over a year.

If enough drug enters the general circulation, alpha-2 agonists also may lower blood pressure, cause sleepiness and tiredness and even depression. These effects can be marked in children, making them totally unsuitable for any child under 20 kg body weight; they should be used with great caution even in larger/older children.

Our most powerful pressure-reducing medications are the **prostaglandin analogues**, latanoprost (Xalatan), travoprost (Travatan), bimatoprost (Lumigan) and tafluprost (Saflutan). They came into use from 1998 onwards and represented the greatest single advance in glaucoma medical management. Needing to be used just once daily, they greatly improved convenience for glaucoma sufferers. As well as separate preparations, the prostaglandin agents are available as fixed combinations with latanoprost (XalaCom), travoprost (DuoTrav) and bimatoprost (GanFort).

Local effects include luscious eye lashes (longer, thicker, darker – some people love this effect), darkening of the eyelid skin, darkening of the eye colour (more common in those with hazel-coloured eyes to start with), redness of the eye surface and eyelid margins and occasionally with longer-term use, some sinking in of the eyes as the fat pads behind the eyeballs shrink.

And finally, there is the family of **miotics**: pilocarpine and carbachol. In one form or another, they were the very first drugs available to reduce eye pressure - back in the 1860s. They enhance outflow through the conventional or trabecular pathways and may be very effective. The reasons they are used relatively infrequently nowadays is because they need to be instilled at least twice daily (they work best if used four times daily) and they cause significant side effects locally.

The miotics tighten the circular muscles inside the eye, stretching and opening the drain tissues to help outflow. In doing so they make the vision blurry and just as it is clearing, it is time for the next drop. They also shrink the pupil allowing less light into the eye, so everything appears dim and dark and it can take a long time for a person to adjust when walking from brightly to dimly lit places (e.g., going into a cinema). In stimulating the inside muscles to contract, the miotics can also give a sensation of tightness or 'pressure' or even pain and headache around the eye. No wonder they are not popular!

As if all this was not bad enough, the miotics can provoke an allergy, may sting, may accelerate cataract formation and then make cataract surgery more

4. Glaucoma treatment

challenging (because the chronically shrunken pupil won't dilate properly for the operation). Especially in short-sighted patients, they increase the risk of retinal detachment.

When one drug is insufficient to reduce IOP to levels thought to be safe, we need combinations of agents that work differently from one another. There is no point in using at the same time two different drugs from the same family: if you do, there is no improved pressure response but a higher chance of side effects. Drugs that lower eye pressure by decreasing inflow (and the various families do this differently from one another) or improving outflow, allow the drugs to complement one another and to benefit your pressure control.

While most of the drugs need to be used twice daily, the prostaglandins do not: once daily gives their maximum benefit and if you instil them twice daily, besides possibly causing more side effects, they work less strongly. So do not overuse them in the hope they will work better!

Although maximum benefit from a drug is usually after about two hours, with the prostaglandins, it is about eight hours later: they take longer 'to kick in'. So, when is the best time to put in once daily drops? The answer is: 'when you remember best'. Some people are 'morning' people and collapse at night, often forgetting their drops because they are too tired; if this is you, use them in the morning. Others are slow or late starters in the mornings or find the early part of the day too rushed to remember drops reliably; if this describes you, please use them at night.

Drops do not have to be used at exactly the same time each day; that would prove impossible for almost everyone. Try to link them with landmarks in your day, such as after waking, when shaving, with breakfast or dinner, when brushing teeth or when retiring to bed. Do whatever works best for you. Remember: drops do not work for those who do not use them. They cannot lower your eye pressure if they are in the bottle and not in your eye. If remembering your drops is a challenge, recognize the problem and talk to your ophthalmologist. You might benefit from an alternative approach to make your vision safe, such as laser techniques.

Your ophthalmologist is your ally against glaucoma. It is the disease that will try to blind you. Get your ophthalmologist to help you to make best use of your eye drops, or consider other treatments.

4. Glaucoma treatment

4.2 Treatment strategies beyond medicines: incisional and non-incisional surgery

Non-incisional laser trabeculoplasty with Argon, Diode or Selective wavelength lasers have been recommended to patients traditionally when medications fail to lower eye pressures to target levels and thus fail to arrest progressive glaucoma damage (when it is an add-on treatment to continued eye drop use) or when medications provoke unacceptable side effects or have been too onerous for patients to use reliably. Because Selective Laser Trabeculoplasty (SLT)(Figure 22) in particular has proven to be relatively effective and to have very few complications, it is increasingly being offered to patients as a viable option at every treatment cross-roads: when treatment is started instead of drops

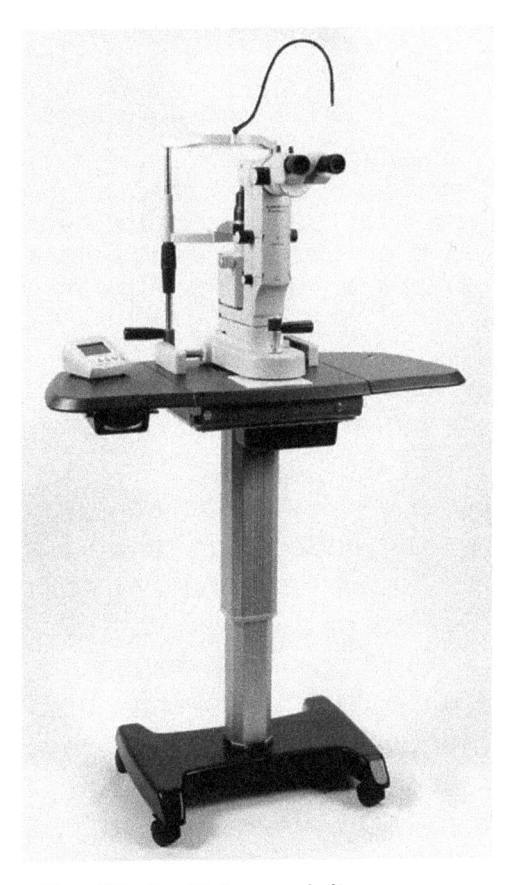

Fig. 22. A slit lamp delivery system for Selective Laser Trabeculoplasty.

73

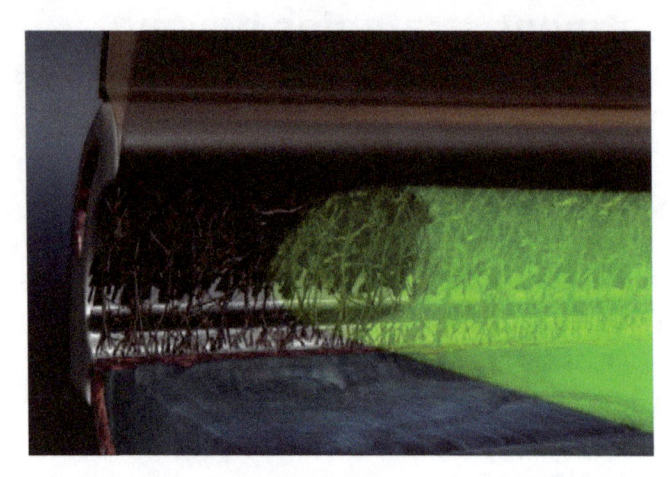

Fig. 23. Diagrammatic representation of application spot of laser light energy to the trabecular meshwork (outflow drain). The laser spot covers the entire 0.4-0.5-mm width of the meshwork. Spots are placed sequentially one alongside the other so that the entire internal surface of the meshwork receives laser energy.

or when treatment needs to be accelerated instead of a second or third or fourth medication.

Laser energy is applied carefully to the inside surface of the trabecular meshwork as a series of spots (Figure 23). Some ophthalmologists routinely treat all 360 degrees of the meshwork with any one use of the laser, either in one or two sessions, whereas others treat a proportion of the meshwork (usually 180 degrees), then wait for four to six weeks to assess the pressure response before proceeding with a second 180-degree treatment if necessary to reduce pressure.

Generally, laser treatment is painless and performed with a couple of drops of topical anaesthetic, the patient seated at a slit lamp through which the laser light

4. Glaucoma treatment

energy is delivered. There is a small chance of slight inflammation for a few days afterwards with some redness, irritability and perhaps sensitivity to light. This abates spontaneously or an anti-inflammatory drop could be used for a few days if necessary. As there is a very small chance that pressure may increase after laser trabeculoplasty with some laser light wavelengths, it is not always 100% trouble-free.

About 75% of patients respond with at least a 20% fall in IOP and about 50% of those who do respond, are still showing benefit five years later. When the pressure reduction abates eventually, SLT seems able to be repeated with almost as good a chance of success as with the first treatment and with no greater risk of complications. As this pressure reduction can be quite modest, if pressures are very high and visual damage is severe (and especially if it is approaching the centre of fixation), sometimes this strategy is by-passed and incisional surgery is recommended sooner.

Open-angle glaucomas associated with pigment dispersion syndrome or pseudo-exfoliation are more likely to respond than primary open-angle glaucoma, but when pressures subsequently rise again, they can do so quite dramatically. This means a person should not be reassured falsely about a good response to laser into thinking they've been 'cured'. Glaucoma is like the ocean: one never knows when the next big wave will come through; one never knows when the condition jumps to another level of aggressiveness. Eternal vigilance with regular monitoring is vital for visual safety.

Another form of laser treatment is relevant for patients with angle-closure: laser peripheral iridotomy is where laser energy vaporizes a small amount of the coloured iris tissue to make a hole through it (Figure 24). This allows aqueous to by-pass the pupil and to take a short cut from behind the iris where it is pumped into the eye to the front of the iris where it drains back to the blood stream. In eyes with angle-closure, such an opening allows the iris to drop backwards away from the

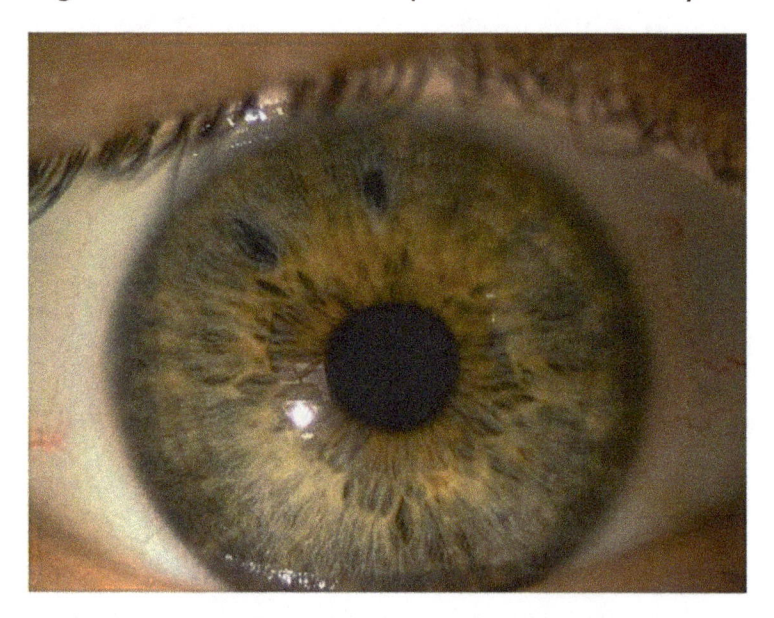

Fig. 24. Two laser peripheral iridotomies have been created through the iris (coloured part of the eye). Ideally, these should be slightly more peripheral than shown here, to minimize the chance of glare problems from light entering the eye through the new openings. These holes through the iris allow aqueous being pumped into the eye by the ciliary body behind the iris, to pass through like a short-cut into the anterior chamber, in front of the iris, without having to go through the pupil in the centre.

4. Glaucoma treatment

trabeculum, allowing it to remain accessible and to avoid injury from repeated contact with the iris. In this way, eye pressures are less likely to increase over the years from accumulated drain damage.

If iridotomy fails to open a partly closed drain adequately, Argon laser peripheral iridoplasty contracts patches of the outer part of the iris, physically pulling it away from the drain (Figure 25).

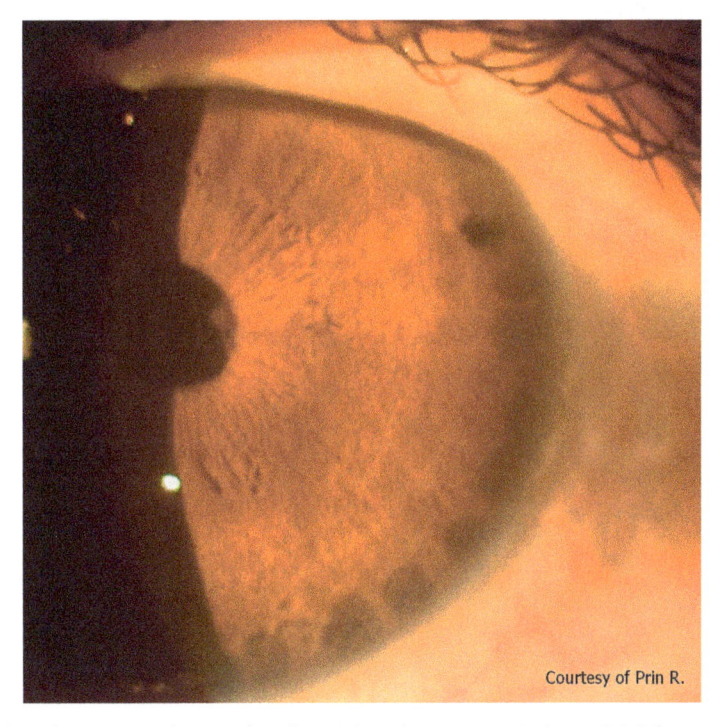

Courtesy of Prin R.

Fig. 25. This eye shows both a Yag-laser peripheral iridotomy and several Argon-laser peripheral iridoplasty marks, which by contracting the iris tissue, push it backwards, away from the trabecular meshwork drain. The meshwork lies like a ring just behind the junction between the clear cornea and the white wall of the eyeball, the sclera.

So, the laser treatment for primary open-angle glaucoma is called trabeculoplasty, while for primary angle closure there are two procedures that may be used depending on the clinical findings: iridotomy and iridoplasty.

Incisional surgery sets out to create a channel bypass for aqueous fluid to exit the eye back to the blood stream without having to pass through either natural outflow pathway. If it succeeds, IOP may be able to be controlled stably for many years at low levels, offering maximal visual safety. As this channel created surgically is not natural, the body's reaction is to heal it: to heal the channel is to seal it and the pressures increase once more.

Therefore, during the operation and sometimes for up to about four weeks afterwards, the ophthalmologist uses anti-cancer agents (mitomycin-C and/or 5-fluoro-uracil) to discourage normal cells from growing and dividing and laying down scar tissue to close the channel. It is like walking a tightrope: the balance is between allowing the surface tissues to heal as they must and yet to discourage the deeper channel through the wall of the eyeball from closing.

There is a second balancing act the patient and the ophthalmologist must go through during those critical post-operative weeks: keeping the fluid flowing through the drain fast enough to keep the pressures low and safe, but not too fast. The eye needs to have some pressure to focus light properly and to see: if the pressure is too low, the vision suffers. Therefore, the

4. Glaucoma treatment

first four weeks post-glaucoma surgery are as important as the operation itself to try to obtain a good result.

Because of these challenges, glaucoma surgery is not entirely predictable. Add to that the small risk of bleeding, of infection and of cataract formation and you can understand why ophthalmologists only consider recommending such surgery to a patient if the risk of not doing the operation exceeds the risk of doing it.

Scarring of the channels is the major cause of failure in glaucoma surgery. The risk of this occurring increases if the eye has undergone previous surgery, especially previous glaucoma surgery (excluding uneventful modern cataract surgery, which does not leave scars in the tissues being operated on in glaucoma). In eyes in this situation, more anti-scarring medication might be needed during and after the operation, along with more powerful and/or more frequent anti-inflammatory medications.

Sometimes fluid flow through the channel is too slow; loosening or removing or cutting (by laser) the stitches that hold the channel partly closed may become necessary.

However, IOP should not be too low. If it is (hypotony), fluid can collect at the back of the eye, causing blurring or shadows in the vision. To focus accurately and to work properly, the eye needs a certain amount of pressure. It should not be too high either.

If scarring of the channels starts to occur, your

ophthalmologist might, in addition, perform under topical anaesthetic (eye drops only) a needle sweep. This involves sweeping a very fine needle through the scar tissue, breaking it up and allowing the fluid to flow more rapidly and more broadly. More 5-fluoro-uracil or mitomycin-C might be necessary with this and for a while afterwards to try to inhibit re-scarring. Very occasionally the surgically created outflow channel is blocked on the inside. Sometimes this is able to be cleared with Yag laser treatment

What does all this mean? Glaucoma drainage surgery consists of two equally important treatment strategies: firstly an operation that is technically meticulous and secondly very careful and often intensive care in the four-to-six-week period after the surgery. Through all this, vision may be quite blurred and variably blurred. Your ophthalmologist will guide you through this with great attention to detail.

If all goes well, your eye ends up with a 'bleb'. This is a kind of 'blister' at the top of the coloured part of your eye, under the upper eyelid, in the white tissues. It represents swelling of those tissues by the fluid emerging from the created channel and being drained back into the blood vessels of the surrounding tissues. These tissues were not designed by evolution to drain fluid, so they swell as they perform their new role.

4.2.1. Possible complications

Besides failure to drain properly (and thus rising IOP), blurring of vision, astigmatism, a drooping of the upper lid (ptosis), foreign-body sensation and other surface eye irritation are all possible after glaucoma surgery. Irritation and the 'it feels like something is in my eye' sensation may be from surface stitches that your body will dissolve over a few weeks or that your ophthalmologist will remove when it is safe to do so, or from decreased lubrication and thus reduced protection of the front surface of your eye by your tear film. Lubricant drops can make a real difference to comfort.

Very occasionally, the created bleb becomes too large or too high and/or might extend downwards over the front surface of your eye (over the cornea). This might require surgical revision.

Severe and possibly sight-threatening complications include infection (endophthalmitis), bleeding into the eye (intra-ocular haemorrhage) and so-called malignant glaucoma (ciliary block glaucoma). These require special treatment, urgently.

While conjunctivitis ('pink eye') in a non-operated eye is usually self-limiting and not harmful, in a patient with a functioning channel through the wall of their eyeball (which results from successful glaucoma drainage surgery) an infection in the tissues outside the eyeball can spread rapidly through the channel and cause a sight-threatening infection within. It is critical

to be seen by your ophthalmologist or someone in his/her place should your eye become red and irritable, especially with a yellowy pus discharge and eyelid stickiness, particularly when you awake in the mornings. Such a risk of infection spreading into the eye is life-long after successful glaucoma drainage surgery.

'Malignant' glaucoma has nothing to do with cancer. It was called by this name because there was no effective treatment for it for a long time. Now that it is known to be related to ciliary block, treatment can be very effective. It results from the aqueous fluid flowing backwards, not forwards in an eye and becoming trapped within or behind the vitreous gel that fills the bulk of an eye's volume, between the retina behind and the focusing lens and ciliary body in front. The swollen vitreous gel or a pocket of aqueous trapped in the gel pushes against the lens and ciliary body and pushes everything forward, collapsing the front chamber (anterior chamber) of the eye. Pressure can rise to very high levels quickly and cause a great deal of pain and damage to sight. While atropine and steroid drops might break the process, allowing everything to return to normal, sometimes laser to break the front surface of the vitreous or even surgery to remove the gel, with or without removal of the focusing lens as well, might become necessary.

There are many variations of glaucoma surgery, most of which are relatively experimental and have not been proven to be effective in the long-term. Some seem to work best when combined with cataract surgery.

4. Glaucoma treatment

However, cataract surgery by itself, without any glaucoma procedure, has been shown to be helpful to reduce IOP in many eyes. Time and careful research will guide your ophthalmologist as to which kind of glaucoma surgery is most likely to help you and to be safest for you, given your special circumstances.

One variation of the trabeculectomy technique uses a stainless steel stent, the *ExPRESS©*. This stent links the partly made channel through to the anterior chamber. This means flow is less likely to be too fast, but the same problems with scarring of the outer part of the wall channel apply as for conventional trabeculectomy.

Newer techniques, all currently under intense investigation, include the Glaukos *iStent* and the Ivantis *Hydrus*, both of which shunt aqueous from the anterior chamber into Schlemm's canal (Figure 4), by-passing the resistance to outflow offered by the trabecular meshwork. It is this meshwork that might offer the greatest obstacle to outflow through the conventional pathway. These are performed as an extension of cataract surgery.

Another approach is *canaloplasty*, in which a channel is created through most of the eyeball wall to open Schlemm's canal into which is passed through its entire circle a special stitch. This is then tied to exert inward pressure on the meshwork. Yet another is *Trabectome©*, in which the trabecular meshwork is cauterized away completely through a segment of its course from inside the eye.

A totally different drainage concept uses devices (*ciliary shunts*, such as the gold shunt) to allow aqueous from the anterior chamber to flow to the potential space between the inside of the eyeball wall and the outside of the choroid layer adjacent to the retina. Normally this potential space is closed as the eye pressure holds the retina and choroid against the inside surface of the eyeball wall. Aqueous shunted in this way subsequently flow through the wall of the eyeball into the orbit socket in which the eye is placed and from there back to the lymphatic and blood vessels.

One of the major disincentives for all these devices is the increased costs they bring to drainage surgery, costs which would be worthwhile bearing if predictable effectiveness, long-term success and safety were to be proven.

One type of drainage surgery that has become popular in certain countries as an alternative to trabeculectomy is **non-penetrating glaucoma drainage surgery (NPGDS)**. These techniques involve creating a channel through the wall of the eyeball, but not 'through-and-through': a thin membrane is left untouched to act as a resistor to aqueous flow. This is hoped to reduce the chances of hypotony through flow that is too rapid and to reduce the chances of infection spreading from the tissues outside the eye to those inside.

As generally NPGDS lowers eye pressures well, but not as much as a successful trabeculectomy, it might not be an option when lower IOP is necessary for visual safety.

Glaucoma drainage devices (GDDs) of a different sort have been available for decades and have been proven to work well – especially in selected cases. These GDDs consist of variations of a soft plastic tube that drains aqueous from the anterior chamber to the outside of the eyeball wall where it flows over a broad firmer plastic surface; from this 'reservoir' it is reabsorbed into surrounding tissues, lymphatics and blood vessels. They go by the names of their inventors: Molteno, Ahmed, Krupin, Baerveldt and Susanna GDDs with design variations to try to improve pressure control long-term and to facilitate insertion. The plate(s) and tube are covered carefully and positioned under the upper eyelid so they are usually not visible unless the eyelid is lifted by fingers.

The tube prevents scarring in the channel through the eyeball wall and the plate(s) try to minimize impact of scarring on the wall surface by providing a large surface area for re-absorption of aqueous.

GDDs have been shown to be highly effective in some forms of glaucoma in which trabeculectomy tends to fail, such as neovascular glaucoma (which may follow retinal vein occlusions or advanced diabetic eye disease), inflammatory glaucoma and glaucoma after a corneal graft. Like all glaucoma surgery, long-term results are not as good as short-term results, but they can be long-lasting.

Following a GDD insertion, generally trabeculectomy is no longer feasible, whereas a GDD is possible after one or more trabeculectomies; because of this, many ophthalmologists reserve GDDs for eyes in which other techniques, including trabeculectomy, have failed.

Cyclodestructive procedures are employed when eye pressure is unlikely to be controlled by improving outflow. Instead the ciliary body, which pumps the aqueous into the eye, is damaged deliberately in a controlled manner to slow the rate of inflow. It's like turning down the tap if the water level in the basin is too high, to allow the drain to cope better. It can be done by freezing or laser techniques, the latter causing less inflammation and thus less discomfort once the local anaesthetic wears off. The laser energy can be applied from the outside or by special techniques from the inside.

Unfortunately, the pressure response is less predictable: often the procedure needs to be repeated. The ophthalmologist tries very hard to avoid over-treating as excess damage to the ciliary body leads to hypotony, from which the eye might never recover. One real possibility is an eye that becomes too soft and shrinks, becoming not only blind, but also potentially unsightly (phthisis).

Even if treatment is optimal, there is a significant chance of reduction in sight. Because of this, cyclo-destructive procedures tend to be performed in eyes with no or very little vision, to keep them comfortable.

4. Glaucoma treatment

Focal Points

- Remember that myths are unproven or false beliefs.

- In glaucoma the most common myths include:

    1. All glaucoma patients have high eye pressures.

    2. Because my vision is good, I can't have glaucoma.

    3. Lifestyle has no influence on glaucoma.

    4. Glaucoma examinations and consultations are tiring and boring (and unnecessary).

    5. If my pressure is less than 21 mm Hg, I'm safe.

    6. There are only a few options in glaucoma treatment.

5. Most common myths in glaucoma

5.1 Myth 1: All glaucoma patients have high eye pressures

When a population is measured, there is a range of eye pressures into which most members fit. In Caucasian communities, the average found is usually around 15 mm Hg with 95% falling between 10 and 20 mm Hg. This range is what is regarded as 'usual' or 'normal' for that group of people.

Definitions of glaucoma until the 1980s included 'eye pressure above normal'.

This was confronted by two inconvenient truths: firstly that depending on country, a large proportion of glaucoma sufferers do not show a raised IOP (one-third in Australia, 80% in Korea, 90% in Japan) and secondly that there are more individuals with IOP greater than 'usual' without glaucoma than there are folks with IOP greater than 'normal' with glaucoma.

Individuals with elevated IOP but no discernible structural or functional damage are regarded as 'ocular hypertensives' with increased risk of developing glaucoma. Eyes with 'usual' IOP with disc and/or visual field damage are diagnosed as having glaucoma and are sometimes sub-diagnosed as having 'normal-pressure' glaucoma. Although eye pressures lie within the normal range these patients also benefit when their IOP is reduced. This is not a different kind of glaucoma from the entire spectrum of primary open-angle glaucoma.

Always ask your ophthalmologist about your optic nerve and visual fields, not just your eye pressure!

5.2 Myth 2: Because my vision is good, I cannot have glaucoma

Cover one eye completely. With the other, look around you. You are totally unaware that even with normal vision, there is an area in your visual field in which you cannot tell the difference between the bottom of a coal mine and the middle of a nuclear explosion: it is your so-called physiological (normal) blind spot; it is the projection into space of your optic disc, which has no photo-receptors and cannot see. Why are we not aware of this hole in our sight? Because we do not see it as a gaping hole. Not only does the other eye fill in the details (the two normal blind spots do not overlap) but even more importantly, the brain paints in the missing details from surrounding clues.

The same thing happens if vision is damaged by glaucoma or even stroke. It is only when the damage is sufficiently extensive for the brain to make mistakes that we start to fall over things, trip on stairs we did not see, knock into people on the side we did not know were there. This has huge implications for safe mobility, independent living and working and driving.

With current technologies, visual loss from glaucoma is irreversible. Stem cell research might change that, but how long it will take to develop effective and safe treatment is an open question. Visual loss from glaucoma tends to be progressive unless treatment arrests it. This means early diagnosis and effective management are vital to keep people visually safe.

It is the side vision that is destroyed in glaucoma, which for the reasons above, you do not miss until it is advanced. The vision used to read, write, recognize faces, watch TV, which would be missed immediately if it were to be damaged, is spared until late in glaucoma.

Testing your side vision yourself is very difficult to do accurately. Have a try if you like and compare the results with your visual field assessments. With a few exceptions, it is impossible to get it right.

What this all means, therefore, is that you cannot reliably judge yourself how much damage this sneaky disease has caused to your sight, or tell accurately whether that damage is stable (treatment is protecting you) or getting worse.

5.3 Myth 3: Lifestyle has no influence on glaucoma

Aerobic exercises (swimming, jogging, cycling, rowing) for at least 30 minutes three times weekly can help to reduce your eye pressures. Such activities also improve your blood pressure and cholesterol, your weight control and your sugar metabolism, all of which help to keep the little blood vessels at the back of your eyes around your optic nerves healthier.

Avoid head-down yoga-type positions as this increases eye pressure, and musicians who play wind instruments might need to discuss this with their ophthalmologist. All these activities can increase eye pressure. They also increase pressure around the brain, however, which might protect the optic nerves from the effects of the raised eye pressures, so we do not know whether or not people need to consider stopping such activities.

If you swim with goggles, ensure they are large enough to sit against the bones of your face and NOT against your eyeballs; if goggles push against the eyes, they increase their pressure, sometimes dramatically.

Another possible cause of high eye pressure is tying a necktie too tightly. This might hinder the flow of blood in the neck veins returning blood from the head, brain and eyes to the heart and as the eyes drain into these veins (they are 'upstream' from them), any rise in vein pressure will increase eye pressure. So avoid wearing shirts or blouses whose collars are too tight for you or tying neckties too tightly.

When you are sleeping or simply lying down, you are horizontal. Lying supine (on your back, facing the ceiling) increases eye pressure because the eyes become level with the heart; compare this with sitting or standing positions where gravity helps blood flow down to the heart and lowers the pressure in the veins of the head, into which the eyes are draining. This is normal and cannot be avoided. However, it is made worse if you lie prone (chest downwards) with your head turned to one side, because it is easy for your eyes to press against the pillows and bedding. Pressure on the eyeball increases IOP and although the pressure slowly equalizes, there is a period when it could be high.

Ensure therefore that your eyes are not making contact with anything when you sleep and if it is comfortable for you to do so, consider elevating the head of the bed slightly. Propping yourself up on more cushions does not seem to lower eye pressures as much as raising the head of the bed.

Smoking not only can increase eye pressure, but it can lead to damage to the vital small blood vessels around the optic nerves; damage to these blood vessels can make them more vulnerable to glaucoma damage.

Marijuana (tetrahydrocannabinol or THC) decreases eye pressures, but only when used at the level that also affects mental function. Unfortunately, the active

5. Most common myths in glaucoma

ingredients in delta-9 THC that lower IOP have not been able so far to be separated from their effects on mood and thinking, despite much effort!

5.4 Myth 4: Glaucoma examinations and consultations are tiring and boring (and unnecessary)

A typical consultation is not tiring or boring or unnecessary at all! It consists of:

1. Assessing the back of the eye with special attention to the optic disc. Looking at these structures with instruments is complemented by photographs and/or computerized images to help to make the diagnosis in the first place and then to try to ensure that treatment is keeping the nerve structures stable and that progressive damage is not occurring.

2. Measuring the eye pressure to try to understand how this major risk factor for damage onset and/or progression has been affected both by time and by treatment. Sometimes this involves multiple measurements and the use of the water-drinking test to try to detect the peak pressures during the day.

3. Analyzing the sensitivity of vision from the centre out to between 24 and 30 degrees away. This visual field test (perimetry) demands concentration and attention if you want reliable results helpful for your treatment. Appendix 2 outlines how you might be able to work with your ophthalmologist and his/her team to get the very best results from this challenging test. Of all the tests done for you by your ophthalmologist and his/her team, it is the

5. Most common myths in glaucoma

visual fields about which most people complain the most.

All these parts of the assessment are vital if you are to receive the world's best care, which is what you deserve. Changes indicating damage allow treatment to be changed to bring things under control once more.

5.5 Myth 5: If my pressure is less than 21 mmHg, I am safe

Depending on your optic nerve's susceptibility to damage, this could be a dangerous concept.

For those people in whom damage occurred with high pressures (say over 30 mmHg), having a treated pressure in the high teens might be safe. For those where damage occurred with lower IOPs, the targets treatment needs to reach might be less than 15 or even less than 12 mmHg.

Not everyone needs to have IOPs at these very low levels. Generally, lower target pressures are needed if the untreated IOP was not too high to start with or vision damage is worse or if the damage is close to the centre of your sight.

Remember, it is the gap between untreated and treated pressures that is your visual safety margin. It is different for everyone and it might even change for you over time: as we age, our nerves become more vulnerable to damage and IOPs might need to be brought down even lower.

5.6 Myth 6: There are only a few options in glaucoma treatment

Although far from perfect, advances have opened up options only dreamt about even twenty years ago:

1. Medication choices and effectiveness are far better than in the past.

2. Laser techniques are safer and may offer a person long-lasting benefits.

3. Conventional trabeculectomy is safer and more effective than in the past.

4. Many newer surgical techniques are being investigated actively.

There are many advances to anticipate with enthusiasm.

Focal Points

- Pseudoexfoliation Syndrome (PXF) and Pigment Dispersion Syndrome (PDS) are two of the most common secondary open angle glaucomas. While PXF is more common in older people, PDS is more common among younger, mostly men.
Both are caused by abnormal deposits on the drainage system (for PXF the deposits are white flakes, for PDS, granules of dark pigment), which damage the drain and causes high and therefore dangerous IOP spikes and high average IOP. These glaucomas demand closer follow-up compared with primary open angle glaucoma.

- Angle closure and angle closure glaucoma: If you have episodes of headaches (sometimes mis-diagnosed as "migraine") be sure you do not have angle closure or angle closure glaucoma.
With sudden angle closure, an eye becomes red, often with severe pain, blurring of vision, sensations of rainbow rings around lights, maybe even with nausea and vomiting. Headaches only on one side of the head may occur. If not treated promptly and effectively, such an acute angle closure crisis can destroy sight in days.
More commonly, angle closure is intermittent, sometimes with episodic visual blurring and "rainbow" effects with mild discomfort, sometimes even completely without symptoms. Almost all oral medications contra indicated in glaucoma are linked to this type of glaucoma.

- **Glaucoma Associated with Steroid Use**
  If you need to use steroids of any kind (tablets, inhaled sprays, creams, injections, eye drops) use them when you have to, no more and no less. Remember to tell all the doctors looking after you that you're using them and that you have glaucoma. While they can increase IOP in some normal people, they can do so more frequently and more dramatically in patients with glaucoma.

- **Congenital and Juvenile Glaucomas**
  Babies with eyes that are too big or one side is bigger than the other, may have congenital glaucoma Other warning signs include watering eyes (other than normal crying or a blocked tear duct) and abnormal sensitivity to light.
  "Watch out for babies with big eyes that water and who shy away from the light."

- **Glaucoma following blunt trauma**
  Anyone who has had an injury to an eyeball needs regular eye checks by an ophthalmologist for the rest of their lives.

6. Other forms of glaucoma worth knowing about

6.1 Pseudoexfoliation syndrome (PXF) or Exfoliation syndrome (XFS)

Pseudoexfoliation syndrome (PXF) is the most widely-known cause of open-angle glaucoma in the world. While its cause is unknown, genetic research has identified a mutation in a gene called the LOXL-1. It is not a straight-forward story, however, as the change in the gene is actually its natural state in nature. So perhaps the non-PXF variation is the mutation! The more we find out, the more questions seem to emerge, which is why and how scientific knowledge advances, gradually, with much thought and work.

Whatever the underlying cause in the cells, an abnormal material that looks like microscopic dandruff (it is nothing like dandruff, of course) is released in the eye where it circulates with the aqueous fluid and is deposited on all the inside structures in the front of the eye. The deposits on the front surface of the crystalline (focusing) lens of the eye act like sandpaper and rub on the back surface of the coloured part of the eye (the iris), which in turn releases pigment granules also into the aqueous circulation.

Both the PXF and pigment material deposit on the trabecular meshwork (the conventional drain) and both block it and damage its cells so they cannot work

6. Other forms of glaucoma worth knowing about

properly to move aqueous out of the eye. Eye pressure may rise and may do so relatively rapidly and severely. This in turn may damage the optic nerve, causing pseudoexfoliative glaucoma.

The PXF material also becomes deposited on the zonule (see below) and may weaken it over time. This could make cataract surgery (which relies on an inherent zonule strength to remove the cloudy lens safely and to replace it with a clear plastic focusing implant) somewhat more risky. Therefore, in a patient with PXF, not uncommonly, the ophthalmologist recommends cataract surgery a bit earlier than usual, before the cataract becomes too dense and hard in consistency, placing more stress on a possibly weakened zonule.

6.2 Pigment dispersion syndrome (PDS)

Pigment dispersion syndrome (PDS) is a specific gene-linked eye condition that affects primarily young men in their 20s and 30s, who are slightly short-sighted (myopic). In these patients, the outer part of the iris is floppier than it should be; it gets pushed backwards by the pulsatile aqueous circulation where its back surface rubs against the zonule. The zonule is a strong structure. like the spokes of a bicycle wheel, that holds the crystalline (focusing) lens of the eye in place. If there is contact between iris and zonule, pigment granules get rubbed off the back surface of the iris to float in the aqueous, which carries them to the trabecular drain. These granules also get deposited on the front surface of the iris and on the back of the cornea (the front window of the eye). All this produces a characteristic appearance your ophthalmologist can detect with a careful slit lamp (biomicroscope) examination.

Like with PXF, these pigment granules block and damage the conventional drainage pathways, increasing eye pressure and putting the optic nerve at the back of the eye at risk.

Because of the extra pigment in the drain, medications might work less well in both PXF and PDS glaucoma compared with the primary open-angle variety of glaucoma. However, laser trabeculoplasty might have a higher chance of lowering IOP. If a good pressure response to laser subsequently declines (as it usually does eventually), the IOP might jump high rapidly. A

6. Other forms of glaucoma worth knowing about

good response to laser therefore does NOT mean a cure, unfortunately and ongoing careful monitoring is essential for visual safety.

6.3 Angle closure and angle-closure glaucoma

Although not as common as open-angle glaucoma, angle-closure glaucoma causes as much visual disability worldwide. This means it is diagnosed late and often missed, like the open-angle varieties of glaucoma, but is even more aggressive overall as it damages nerve connexions between eye and brain.

Angle closure is particularly common among people of Chinese, Mongolian, Indian and other Asian origin as well as among Inuit. It is found in Caucasians and Africans as well, but less frequently. It starts off as an inherited crowding of structures in the front of the eye: the front chamber is shallow, the iris and lens are further forward than they should be; as a result there is a tight fit between lens and iris.

Aqueous fluid, pumped into the eye at the ciliary body behind the iris, meets higher resistance than it should as it moves between iris and lens and then through the pupil to reach the anterior chamber from where it drains out of the eye through the trabecular meshwork and unconventional pathways. This increased resistance means there is a pressure difference between the chamber behind the iris compared with the chamber in front and this pressure difference pushes the iris further forwards – into what is already a shallow space.

This push from behind can press the outside part of the iris against the trabecular meshwork, physically blocking it and damaging it, so that even when the iris

6. Other forms of glaucoma worth knowing about

intermittently drops back, the drain does not work as well as it should.

Because the focusing lens of the eye grows like a tree-trunk throughout life, this inherited structural problem gets worse with increasing age (as do so many things in life). The increasing volume of the lens crowds everything around it and presses ever tighter against the back of the iris, which in turn is pressed more strongly and more often against the drain.

Should the drain suddenly close (like putting a plug into the basin while the water is running in through the tap: the water level rises) the aqueous fluid, which is still being pumped into the eye, has nowhere to go and the eyeball pressure rises rapidly. This causes redness of the eye, often severe pain, blurring of vision, sensations of coloured rainbow rings around lights, maybe even nausea and vomiting. The person feels very ill. This is a full-blown acute angle closure crisis, which can destroy sight in a day or two (Figure 26).

Fortunately, this occurs rather infrequently and with the severe symptoms, the person usually seeks help relatively quickly. The sooner treatment can be started, the better the outlook not only to save sight, but also to restore normal function later.

More commonly, angle closure is intermittent and self-resolving, sometimes with episodic visual blurring and 'rainbow' effects with mild discomfort, sometimes completely without symptoms. This is the really dangerous form of angle closure: the drain becomes

Glaucoma: How to Save Your Sight!

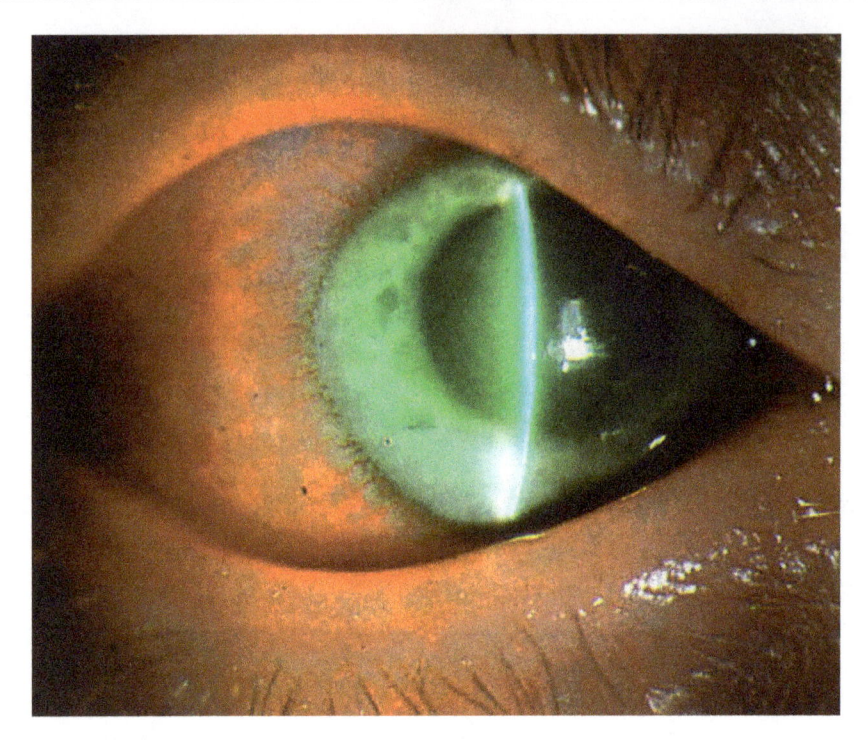

Fig. 26. An eye suffering an acute angle closure crisis. Note the redness, the cloudiness of the cornea and the semi-dilated and fixed-size pupil. The patient felt ill and suffered severe pain in and around the eye along with blurred vision and coloured rings around lights.

progressively damaged and scarred (so it will never be able to work properly again), eye pressures rise slowly and permanently with optic nerve and visual damage.

An eye examination allows the shallow anterior chamber to be detected and the narrowed, maybe damaged drain to be identified (with a special mirror called a gonioscopy lens, used on the slit lamp)(Figures 15 & 16). This is in addition to measuring the pressure, assessing the optic nerve structure and visual field results.

6. Other forms of glaucoma worth knowing about

If angle closure is identified, or if a person has narrow drains that might close (and there are ways to highlight those at greater risk), a preventative laser peripheral iridotomy usually opens the drain more widely and improves access of the aqueous to the trabecular meshwork. This is a little hole drilled through the outer part of the iris and it works by creating a short-cut for the aqueous to flow from behind to in front of the iris, without having to push its way between the iris and the lens to get through the pupil (Figures 24 & 25). This means there is no longer a pressure difference between the chambers behind and in front of the iris and therefore no added pressure pushing the iris forwards onto the drain tissues.

The person's underlying structure of a shallow anterior chamber remains, of course and sometimes this measure does not protect the drain long-term as the lens continues to grow and may physically push the iris onto the drain. Removing the lens eliminates the problem; where there is a cataract (see below), the decision to go ahead with cataract surgery becomes easier. Where there is no cataract, removing a 'clear' lens is more controversial, but sometimes is in the best interest of the patient.

There is another laser procedure that might help if the iridotomy is insufficient: Argon laser peripheral iridoplasty, which uses the laser to contract the outer part of the iris away from the drain (Figure 25). This may either work really well or prove disappointing: every eye is different. If it works, it may need to be repeated after a few years.

After an acute crisis has been resolved and sometimes after a peripheral iridotomy or iridoplasty, ongoing anti-glaucoma medications are necessary to keep the pressure under control, to keep sight safe; this is the case if the outflow pathways have been damaged before treatment was performed.

Angle closure and angle-closure glaucoma usually affect both eyes, although, as with the open-angle glaucomas, often one eye is more affected than the other. Both need treatment. If only one eye is affected, your ophthalmologist will be looking very hard to find a specific cause for it in that eye.

There are a number of medications that might precipitate an attack of angle closure, such as decongestants used for coughs and colds, some treatments for bladder problems and some anti-depressants. They have warnings in their consumer information sheets. They should have no effects on eyes with open-angle glaucoma.

6. Other forms of glaucoma worth knowing about

6.4 Glaucoma associated with steroid use

What might increase the eye pressure in all kinds of glaucoma are the powerful drugs known as steroids. These include prednisone, prednisolone, cortisone, hydrocortisone, betamethasone and dexamethasone. There are many more.

They are used mostly for serious conditions, but also sometimes might be recommended for relatively minor conditions. If a person has to use them (such as for general inflammatory diseases or for arthritic pain relief or asthma control) make sure your ophthalmologist knows about it. Over time, but sometimes quite quickly, they can push up IOP, especially if used as eye drops for certain eye conditions! A good general rule is: if you need to use steroids of any kind (tablets, inhaled sprays, creams, injections, eye drops) use them when you have to, no more and no less. Do not over-use them or use them flippantly – and remember to tell all the doctors looking after you that you are using them and that you have glaucoma.

6.5 Neovascular ('new vessel') glaucoma

Some eyes can suffer from a lack of oxygen. This might happen because: (1) the main artery on one side of the neck (the carotid) becomes blocked and insufficient nutrients are delivered to the eye on that side; (2) because diabetes damages the small blood vessels (the capillaries) in the retina, damaging their ability to supply the retina; (3) because the retinal vein becomes occluded and blood supply to the retina becomes seriously affected.

In these circumstances, the retina releases emergency molecules to try to create new blood vessels to deliver more supplies. This produces a myriad of new, abnormal blood vessels in both the back and the front of the eye. These little vessels do not function normally, they leak large molecules into the eye creating havoc and formation of scar tissue which contracts and disrupts normal eye structure. Aqueous flow becomes blocked in several possible ways, including at the drain. IOP rises dramatically, the eye becomes ever more red and painful and vision often is damaged badly.

Treatment is to try to fix the cause if possible, to stop the release of emergency molecules with laser, to control inflammation with steroids and sometimes atropine, and to stop abnormal blood vessel formation with intra-ocular injections of anti-VEGf medicines such as Lucentis©, Avastin© or Eylea. Often, raised IOP cannot be controlled with medications or laser, so surgery becomes necessary, if visual potential justifies it. In this case, usually a glaucoma drainage device

6. Other forms of glaucoma worth knowing about

is used. If there is insufficient vision to justify such surgery, cyclodestruction might be used to control pain.

6.6 Juvenile or congenital glaucoma

Affecting about one baby in 10,000 births and in 75% of cases bilateral, babies can suffer from glaucoma, which results from abnormal development of their outflow drains. Sometimes, the eye pressure is markedly increased even before or shortly after birth, or they can become elevated during infancy, childhood or adolescence. Usually, the younger the person is when the trouble begins, the more severe the outflow abnormalities and the worse the glaucoma.

In babies and very young children, the eyeball is stretchable; high pressures therefore make the eye expand. Relative to their head and body size, babies normally have eyes that are larger than adults; but if the eyes are too big, that could be a warning sign. Abnormally big eyes are called 'buphthalmic' ('ox-like').

Other warning signs include watering eyes (other than from normal crying of course, or a blocked tear duct) and sensitivity to light. Pay special attention to babies with big, watering eyes who shy away from the light!

If the stretching of the eyeball reaches a critical point, a membrane inside the cornea (window of the eye) may split and the normally clear cornea (which gives the normal eye its lustre) becomes white and cloudy. This can happen suddenly and means that the baby needs to be seen by a pediatric ophthalmologist as quickly as possible.

Treatment might involve medicines to help prepare

6. Other forms of glaucoma worth knowing about

the eye(s) for surgery, which is what is necessary. Any anti-glaucoma medications need to be used in babies and children with even more care than in adults, as the safety margin for side effects is considerably smaller.

Surgery aims to restore aqueous outflow by opening the partly blocked drainage system or by by-passing it altogether. Goniotomy and trabeculotomy are the two most often used procedures, but sometimes trabeculectomy, a glaucoma drainage device or even cyclodestruction might be necessary. Treatment is more complicated if there are other eye (or general) inherited abnormalities present.

6.7 Glaucoma associated with facial port wine stain

If a person is born with a haemangioma (angiomatosis or port wine stain) involving their face, it means the pressure in the veins behind and around the eye could be elevated. As the eye drains aqueous into these veins (the eye is 'upstream' to the veins), a raised venous pressure leads directly to a raised eye pressure. If the upper eyelid is involved in the stain, the risk of this kind of glaucoma is about 50%.

As most people are unaware of this possible additional problem, we wanted to publicize it so that affected individuals know to have their eyes checked carefully. Early treatment offers real protection from visual damage. A neurological assessment is also necessary, as abnormal blood vessels could lie around the brain as well.

6. Other forms of glaucoma worth knowing about

6.8 Glaucoma following blunt trauma

When a blunt object hits the eyeball hard, it indents it and sends a shock wave through the eye in thousandths of a second. This shockwave can tear and damage internal eye structures, including the trabecular drainage system. If this is damaged, it works less well, sometimes even decades later, with rising eye pressures and glaucoma damage to the optic nerve head. This happens without warning.

Anyone who has had an injury to their eye(s) needs regular eye checks by an ophthalmologist for the rest of their lives if any subsequent glaucoma is to be detected early and efficient treatment offered to safeguard vision.

6.9 Inflammatory eye disease and glaucoma

There are several kinds of inflammation that can affect the eye, causing problems variously labelled as 'iritis' or 'uveitis' which might involve primarily the structures at the front or the back of the eye. Inflammation of the front of the eye is more likely to interfere with aqueous circulation and drainage and therefore more likely to increase eye pressure and provoke glaucoma.

While infections (e.g., tuberculosis, toxoplasmosis and various viruses) can cause this inflammation, often its cause cannot be identified. Another known association in children and adolescents is juvenile arthritis.

Treatment consists of three important principles:

- Try to identify the cause and treat it if possible;

- Bring the inflammation under control as quickly and as effectively as possible;

- Control the eye pressure to protect the optic disc and thus the visual field from glaucoma.

Management of glaucoma associated with inflammatory eye disease can be challenging and requires intense efforts by patient and ophthalmologist.

6. Other forms of glaucoma worth knowing about

Focal Points

- If both cataract and glaucoma surgeries are necessary, they might be combined into one operation or the ophthalmologist might recommend cataract surgery alone; cataract surgery on its own may reduce IOP.

- Preferably, glaucoma surgery should not be performed before planned cataract surgery as the healing process after the cataract operation may lead to failure of the previous glaucoma surgery.

7. Glaucoma and cataract together

As both glaucoma and cataract increase in frequency as people age, they are often found together. Furthermore, both long-term anti-glaucoma medications (especially with benzalkonium chloride preservative) and glaucoma (or other) eye surgery can produce or accelerate cataract formation.

The eye has to focus incoming light onto the retina at the back to generate a clear image. From this, the retina sends nerve impulses (like tiny electric currents) along the optic nerve to the brain for decoding and visual perception. This focus is achieved by the crystalline lens, which has to be clear to transmit and focus the light cleanly. A cloudy lens is what is known as a cataract. It is normal for the crystalline lens to lose its clarity with increasing age.

When that cloudiness produces sufficient blurring ('things are out of clear focus' or 'it's like looking through a dirty spectacle lens') or glare problems (often especially with night driving when headlights of oncoming cars seem to 'spray' outwards) or dimming of vision, then it increasingly affects a person's ability to live and work and function normally. Then it is time to have the cataract removed and replaced by a crystal clear plastic implant.

Because the results of modern cataract surgery are so good, the chances of success are so high (usually about 95-97%) and the recovery is so predictable for otherwise-normal eyes, cataract surgery has become the most common operation of any kind performed in many countries. However, as it is not 100% safe and it is not 100% free from possible problems, it is usually advised only when visual problems justify the small risk of something unwanted happening.

In eyes with glaucoma and glaucoma damage to the vision (or any other eye problems, like macular degeneration or diabetic eye disease, for example), successful cataract surgery can only restore the sight to the level permitted by the other eye diseases. Therefore, it is important to have realistic expectations from any surgical interventions.

If an eye has had successful glaucoma drainage surgery and has a functioning drainage bleb and then develops a cataract that requires surgical extraction, the inflammation that inevitably follows even ideal cataract surgery may kick-start a renewed healing process in the bleb and lead to bleb failure. Intense anti-inflammatory treatment with even more careful follow-up than usual can prevent this from happening and sometimes anti-scarring treatment like 5-fluoro-uracil injections alongside the bleb might be necessary to safeguard ongoing performance.

For these reasons, if both cataract and glaucoma surgeries are necessary, they might be combined into one operation or the ophthalmologist might recommend cataract surgery first in the hope it could benefit pressure control enough

7. Glaucoma and cataract together

to allow glaucoma surgery to be postponed or even deferred indefinitely. Preferably, glaucoma surgery should not be scheduled before planned cataract surgery.

Appendix 1: How to instil eye drops

1. Wash your hands.

2. Take the lid off the bottle and have a clean tissue handy.

3. Sit and lean far back or lie down on your back so you're looking up at the ceiling.

4. Rest the heel of one hand (holding the bottle) on your forehead to steady it.

5. With the other hand, gently pull your lower eye lid down to form a little 'cup'.

6. Position the inverted bottle over your eye and gently squeeze to instil one drop.

7. If you're not sure a drop has gone in properly, instil more till you are certain. (Sometimes it helps to keep the bottle of drops in the fridge to make them cold. That way you can feel them go in very easily.)

8. Do the same at once for the other eye (assuming you need the drops in both eyes).

9. Close your eyes without squeezing or blinking repeatedly.

10. Place the tissue over the eyes to absorb any excess drops that run onto the skin of the lids.

11. Using the pulps of both index fingers, press gently over the tear sac at the nose-corner of the eyes and hold steady pressure with your eyes still closed for at least two and preferably three minutes. This minimizes absorption into the body of the medicines, making them safer, and keeps them longer in the eyes, making them more effective (See Figure 21).

12. If you need a second different drop (or more) remember you must wait at least five minutes between drops so that one doesn't wash out the other. You could wait longer, but not less than five minutes.

13. If you wear contact lenses, wait at least 20 minutes after instilment of the drops before inserting them.

14. If you remember your drops late, instil them when you remember and put the next lot in at the usual time.

15. When you travel, switch your drop timings to the place where you happen to be, even if the interval between drops is temporarily increased or decreased while travelling.

Appendix 2: How to do the best-possible visual field test

1. Make sure you are comfortable at the perimeter:

- Your feet should be placed comfortably so that your thighs are horizontal;

- Your back should be supported;

- Your chin height should be adjusted so your forehead touches the holding band easily;

- Your other eye should be covered comfortably and fully: it could be open or closed as you prefer;

- Your arms should be supported so your shoulders and neck do not tire.

2. These are the instructions you should receive before starting the test:

- 'We are getting you to do this test to give us information. We want to see how full and perfect your vision is or, if it isn't, we want to know where the damage is, and what sort of damage it is.'

- 'The test is not difficult, but to get the best information for your care, it needs to be done in a particular way.'

- 'The key to success is to look straight ahead all the time.'

- 'Let the light come to you – don't go looking for it.'

- 'You won't see the light a good deal of the time, so don't worry if time seems to be passing without a light appearing. The machine makes the light very dim so that it can tell when you can just see it.'

- 'Press the button when you think you see the light. All the lights you see, matter — they can be fuzzy, dim, bright, it doesn't matter.'

- 'Blink whenever you need to, but do so when you press the button. That will stop your eyes drying out and hurting, and you won't miss any lights.'

- 'Hold the button down when you want to rest. That will pause the machine. Release the button when you want to continue. Remember you can rest as often as you like. You're the one controlling the machine; the machine is not running you.'

- If you have never done a visual field test before, you need to have a practice run first. This is called the demonstration programme. Sometimes even people who have done the test previously benefit from a revision test.

3. Support to expect during the test:

- You should not be abandoned during the test: the technician should return regularly and frequently to check you're going satisfactorily;

- You should receive reassurance and encouragement during the test;

- If things are not going well, the technician should try to identify and to rectify the cause of the problem; you should not feel disparaged or 'blamed';

- If you just can't cope, the technician should consider rescheduling the test.

- The technician needs to be patient, more patient, and then even more patient: it is NOT an easy test.

4. The testing environment needs to be quiet to support concentration.

Further reading

Quigley H. Glaucoma: What Every Patient Should Know: A Guide from Dr. Harry Quigley, 2011

Marks E, Montauredes R. Coping with Glaucoma. New York, NY: Avery Publishing Group, 1997.

Wong T. Glaucoma: The Complete Guide. A Patient Handbook. Singapore: Medjay Group, 2011.

About the authors

Ivan Goldberg

Ivan Goldberg is Clinical Associate Professor at the University of Sydney, Head of the Glaucoma Unit, Sydney Eye Hospital and the Director, Eye Associates, Sydney Australia. He has an active interest in patient care, teaching, clinical research and developing professional associations and has authored or co-authored over 150 peer-reviewed papers, 30 Editorials and 30 books or chapters in books.

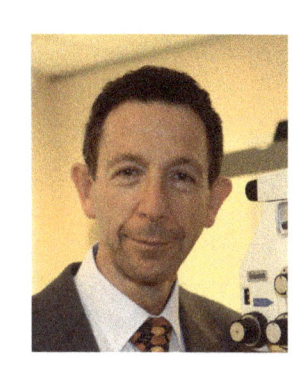

Goldberg is Vice-President and Immediate Past President of Glaucoma Australia. He is Immediate Past President of the Asia Pacific Glaucoma Society and the Australian and New Zealand Glaucoma Interest Group, a past President of the World Glaucoma Association and of the Royal Australian and New Zealand College of Ophthalmologists and is an Active Member of the Glaucoma Research Society.

For his work in glaucoma nationally and internationally, Ivan Goldberg has been honoured with Medal of the Order of Australia, with the International Scholar Award of the American Glaucoma Society, with the Robert Ritch Award of the Glaucoma Foundation of New York, with the Bartisch Medal from the University of Dresden, by the University of Sao Paulo and with honorary memberships of the Philippine and South African Glaucoma Societies.

Remo Susanna Jr.

Remo Susanna is Professor and Chair at the Department of Ophthalmology, Sao Paolo, Brazil, Head of the Glaucoma Service, Past President of the World Glaucoma Association, Founder and Past President of the Latin American Glaucoma Society, and member of the International Committee of ARVO. Member of the Board of Governors of World Glaucoma Association, Active member of the Glaucoma research Society and Von Graeffe society, Past President of Brazilian Glaucoma Society, Past President of the Pan American Glaucoma Society, Past Director of the department of Ophthalmology of Albert Einstein Hospital, São Paulo Brazil.

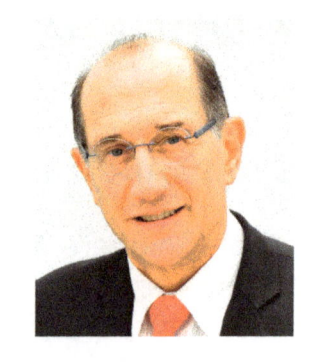

Remo Susanna received the American Academy of Ophthalmology Achievement Award. For lifetime contributions to glaucoma research, education, patient care, and international collaboration, he was given the International Scholar Award. He also received the World Glaucoma Association Award, an award that recognizes extraordinary contributions to the World Glaucoma Association, glaucoma patients and to the global glaucoma community.

Susanna authored or co-authored over 140 peer-reviewed papers, and 13 books and 40 book chapters and has given more than 600 lectures. He is the inventor of the Susanna Glaucoma Implant and the developer of Glaucoma Early Diagnostic Program, EDP. He recently

About the authors

received the Brazilian Award LIDE, for his enormous contributions to the Brazilian people in the field of ophthalmology and glaucoma.

Frequently asked questions

Is there any way to prevent glaucoma?
There is nothing that will prevent glaucoma, but you can slow down its development with early treatment. Therefore, it is very important that you have regular eye exams. Angle closure glaucoma may be avoidable with a timely laser treatment.

If I have glaucoma, will I become blind?
The chances are good that you will not go blind if you take your medication correctly and regularly and follow up with your doctor.

If my parent has glaucoma, will I get it?
Not necessarily, but it does increase your risk. You have approximately 10 times more chance to have glaucoma compared to someone that does not have a glaucoma parent

If drops don't work, will I go blind?
There are many different types of medications (in eye drops or pills) that are used to treat glaucoma. If this doesn't work for you there is the option to perform laser treatment in some cases where the disease in not too far advanced. In this case or if previous treatment failed, several kinds of surgeries can be performed.

Do I need to do visual field tests again?
Early peripheral visual field loss is not noticeable to the patient, and its slow progression makes its recognition nearly impossible without special testing. Although intraocular pressure reduction may reduce or stop the progression of the disease, the only way to be sure that the disease is under control is to confirm no functional progression of the disease with the visual field and structural progression with optic disc assessment with special equipment.

Is there an optic nerve graft or any other way to restore my optic nerve?
Unfortunately, at the present time we are unable to restore an optic nerve. Newer neuroprotective and neurorestoration medicines have been put on trial but once an optic nerve has been damaged, with today's technology the accompanying vision loss is permanent.

Can I use a contact lens after trabeculectomy?
Preferably contact lenses should be avoided after trabeculectomy. Soft lenses increase the risk of infection inside the eye after trabeculectomy fourfold and the results of the infection inside the eye can be devastating. Soft lenses can irritate or rupture the filtration "bleb" that is created during the trabeculectomy procedure, reducing its efficiency.

Frequently asked questions

Can I use Viagra?
Yes you can: there should be no problem from a glaucoma perspective.

Index key words

Age   13
Adherence   54, 56
Angle closure glaucomas   42, 44, 45, 63, 76, 78,
    106-110
Cataract   121-123
Childhood glaucoma   114
Ciliary block   81, 82
Congenital glaucoma   114-115
Corneal thickness   18, 48
Cyclo-destruction   86
Ethnicity   13
Family history   13
Gonioscopy   **42**, 45
How to do visual fields   127-129
Infection   62, 79, 81, 82, 84, 118, 138
Instilling Eye Drops   125-126
    Physical difficulties instilling eye drops   54
    Timing eye drop instillations   56
Juvenile glaucoma   114-115
Laser treatments   11, 19, 23, 45, 58, 61, 73-78, 79, 80,
    82, 86, 98, 104, 105, 109, 112, 137
    Laser trabeculoplasty   61, 73-78, 104,
        Selective   73
        Argon   73
        Diode   73
    Peripheral iridotomy   **76**, 77, 109, 110
    Peripheral iridoplasty   **77**, 109
Lifestyle factors   93-94
Exercise   93
Swimming   93
Sleeping   49, 94

Necktie   93
Smoking   94
Marijuana   94
Malignant glaucoma   81, 82
Medications   63-72
    Alpha-2 agonists   68-69
        Apraclonidine   68, 69
        Brimonidine   68, 69
    Beta-blockers   65-68
        Betaxolol   65, 66
        Timolol   65, 66, 68
    Carbonic anhydrase inhibitors   67-68
        Acetazolamide   67
        Brinzolamide   66, 68, 69
        Dorzolamide   66, 68
    Miotics   70-71
        Pilocarpine   70
    Prostaglandins   71
        Bimatoprost   65, 69
        Latanoprost   65, 69
        Tafluprost   69
        Travoprost   65, 69
Myths about Glaucoma   89- 98
Non-adherence   47, 53-58
Non-persistence   47
Open angle glaucomas   13, 45, 75, 100, 110
Optic Nerve Head   24, 26, 117
Perimetry / Perimeter   26-28, 46, 47, 95, 127
Pressure (IOP)   14, 16, 17, 47, 48- 50, 55, 67, 68, 71, 75, 78, 79, 81, 83, 84, 89, 90, 94, 97, 104, 111, 112
    Target eye pressure   48, 49
Secondary glaucomas   42-43, 63

Index

    Inflammatory   43, 118
    Neovascular   85, 112-113
    Pigment Dispersion   75, **104-105**
    Port wine stain   115
    Pseudoexfoliation   13, **102-103**
    Steroid induced   43, **111**
    Trauma (injury)   117
Seven Sins   13-59
    Failure to diagnose   16-37
    Failure to detect progressive damage   38-41
    Failure to diagnose type of glaucoma   42-45
    Failure to stage disease accurately   46-47
    Insufficient eye pressure reduction   48-50
    Delayed onset of treatment   51-52
    Non-adherence to therapy   53-58
Surgery   19, 47, 58, 61, 62, 70, **73-86**, 103, 112, 113, 115, 121, 122, 123
    Trabeculectomy   **83**, 84, 85, 86, 99, 115, 138
        Express shunt   83
    Canaloplasty   83
        iStent   83
        Hydrus   83
        Gold shunt   84
    Drainage Devices   85-86
        Susanna   85
        Molteno   85
        Ahmed   85
        Baerveldt   85
        Krupin   85
    Non-penetrating   84
Tonometry   17
Visual Fields   29, 38, 39, 40, 90
    Normal   30, 91, 48

Mild damage   32, 40, 48
   Moderate damage   24, 34, 48, 51
   Severe damage   26, 36, 39, 48, 75
Water Drinking Test   **49-50**, 95

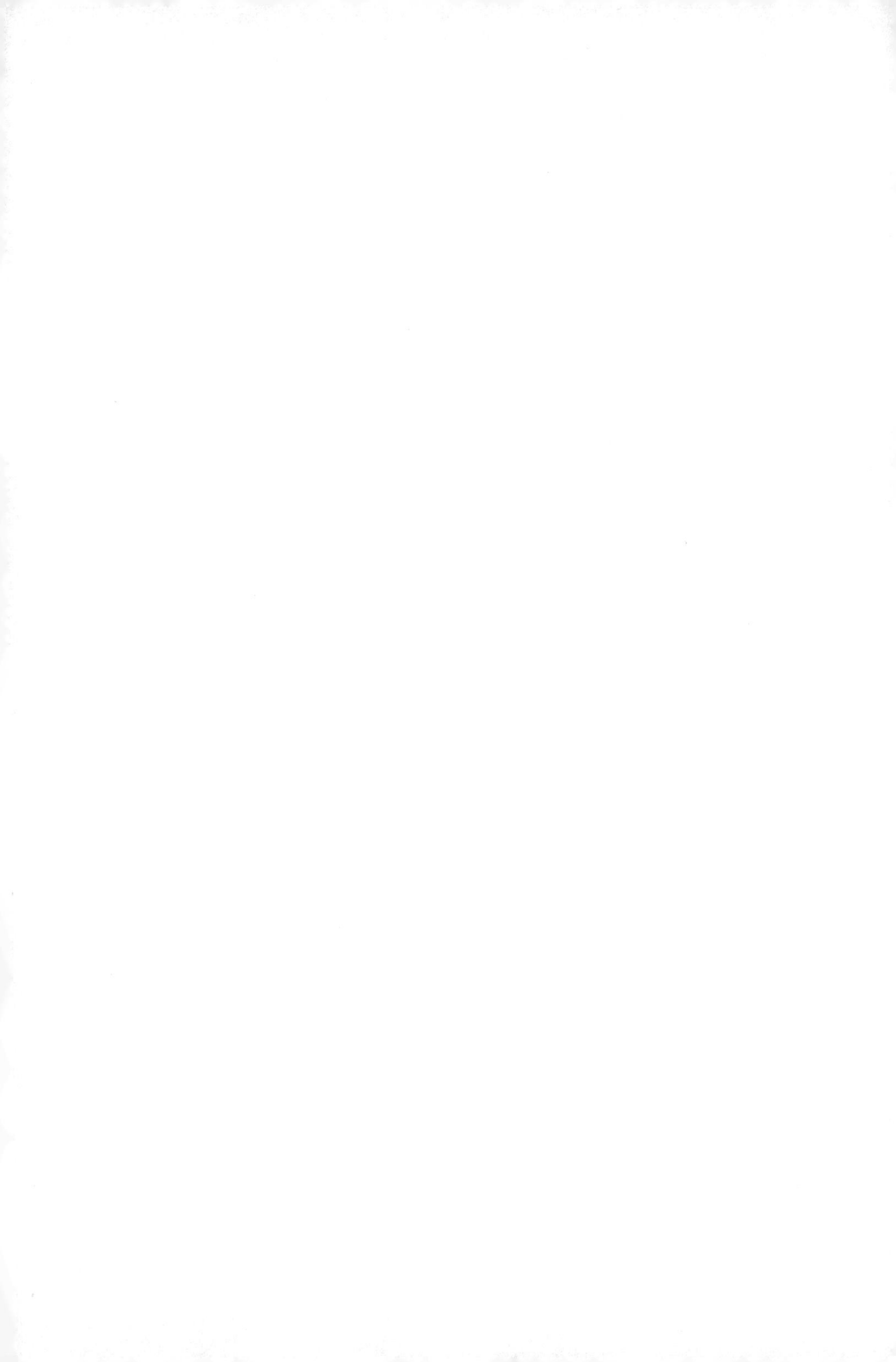